Improving Communication in Mental Health Settings

Improving Communication in Mental Health Settings draws on empirical studies of real-world interactions to demonstrate contemporary practice-based evidence, providing effective strategies for communicating with patients/clients in mental health settings.

The book integrates clinical experience and language-based evidence drawn from qualitative research. Drawing on studies that utilize scientific language-based approaches such as discourse and conversation analysis, it focuses on social interaction between professionals and patients/clients to demonstrate effective communication practices. Chapters are led by clinical professionals and feature a range of mental health settings, different mental health conditions and types of patient/client, and evidence-based recommendations.

This book is an essential guide for professionals working in mental health and/or social work, and those training or working in clinical areas of mental health practice.

Michelle O'Reilly is an associate professor of communication in mental health at the University of Leicester, UK.

Jessica Nina Lester is an associate professor of inquiry methodology in the School of Education at Indiana University, Bloomington, USA.

Improving Communication
in Mental Health Settings

Evidence-Based Recommendations from
Practitioner-led Research

Edited by Michelle O'Reilly and
Jessica Nina Lester

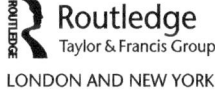

Routledge
Taylor & Francis Group

LONDON AND NEW YORK

First published 2021
by Routledge
52 Vanderbilt Avenue, New York, NY 10017

and by Routledge
2 Park Square, Milton Park, Abingdon, Oxon, OX14 4RN

Routledge is an imprint of the Taylor & Francis Group, an informa business

Library of Congress Cataloging-in-Publication Data
A catalog record for this title has been requested

ISBN: 978-0-367-45606-1 (hbk)
ISBN: 978-0-367-45605-4 (pbk)
ISBN: 978-1-003-02433-0 (ebk)

Typeset in Times New Roman
by MPS Limited, Dehradun

Contents

Acknowledgements

Each of the chapters included in this book were reviewed by both an academic and a practitioner working in the field of mental health. Some of the reviewers hold joint practitioner and academic roles. Such a robust reviewing framework ensured the academic rigor of each chapter and the quality of the evidence presented, but also assured that each chapter would be accessible and useful to practitioners. We are therefore very grateful to the following reviewers who took time out of their busy schedules to review the chapters. We list them here in alphabetical order.

Mohammed Abbas; Consultant Adult Psychiatrist (Leicestershire Partnership NHS Trust) and associate professor (Hon), (University of Leicester)

Amanda Bateman: senior lecturer early childhood (Swansea University)

Aditi Chaudhuri: consultant child and adolescent psychiatrist (Leicestershire Partnership NHS Trust)

Dave Clarke: foundation professor of nursing (University of West England)

Gemma Dacey: neurodevelopmental clinician (Children's Neurodevelopmental Service Coventry and Warwickshire Partnership NHS Trust)

Alice Dolton: specialist learning mentor, overseeing mental and emotional well-being (Aspire Life-skills Learning Centre for young people with diagnoses of ASD)

Stuart Ekberg: senior research fellow (DECRA) (Queensland University of Technology)

Riya George: lecturer in clinical communication skills (Barts and The London School of Medicine and Dentistry)

Elizabeth Hale: clinical and health psychologist (The Dudley Group NHS Foundation Trust)

Valerie Harwood: professor of sociology and anthropology of education (University of Sydney)

Avinash Hiremath: consultant psychiatrist for people with learning disabilities and medical director (Leicestershire Partnership NHS Trust)

Fawzia Kauser: family and systemic psychotherapist (Leicestershire Partnership NHS Trust)

Joyce Lamerichs: assistant professor and senior researcher (VU University, Amsterdam)

Mary Lavelle: senior research fellow in mental health (City, University of London)

Maeuve McColgan: lead family and systemic psychotherapist (Leicestershire Partnership NHS Trust)

Elizabeth McSweeney: general practitioner (Saffron Health)

Elizabeta Mukaetova-Ladinska: professor in psychiatry of old age (University of Leicester and Leicestershire Partnership NHS Trust)

Tom Muskett: senior lecturer and disability liaison officer (Leeds Beckett University)

Kerry Onyejekwe: lecturer in education (University of Leicester)

Janet Smithson: senior lecturer in psychology (University of Exeter)

Trini Stickle: assistant professor (Western Kentucky University)

Tom Strong: professor of family therapy (University of Calgary)

Ali Tempest: associate professor in speech and language therapy (De Montfort University)

Sam Tromans: honorary academic clinical lecturer in social and epidemiological psychiatry (University of Leicester) and adult psychiatrist (Leicestershire Partnership NHS Trust)

Eleftheria Tseliou: associate professor of research methodology and qualitative methods (University of Thessaly)

Ellen Vaughn: associate professor (Indiana University)

Mark Waddington: clinician manager (Director) and psychotherapist for placement support (an adoption support agency working with complex families) (Leicester) and PhD student (University of Leicester)

Editor Biographies

Dr Michelle O'Reilly (**BSc [Hons], MSc, MA, PhD, PGCAPHE**) is an associate professor of communication in mental health at the University of Leicester and a research consultant and quality improvement advisor for Leicestershire Partnership NHS Trust. Michelle is also a chartered psychologist in health. Michelle has research interests in mental health and social media, self-harm and suicidal behaviour, neurodevelopmental conditions, and child mental health services, such as mental health assessments and family therapy. Michelle recently won the Anselm Strauss Award for Qualitative Family Research for her co-authored contribution on discursive psychology in this area (with Nikki Kiyimba and Jessica Lester). Michelle has expertise in qualitative methodologies and specialises in discursive psychology and conversation analysis.

Dr Jessica Nina Lester (**BA, MEd, PhD**) is an associate professor of inquiry methodology in the Department of Counseling & Educational Psychology in the School of Education at Indiana University, Bloomington. Jessica has published over 80 peer-reviewed journal articles, as well as numerous books and book chapters focused on discourse and conversation analysis, disability studies, and more general concerns related to qualitative research. Her co-authored methodological texts include *Doing Qualitative Research in a Digital World; Collecting Naturally Occurring Data; Doing Applied Conversation Analysis: A Practical Guide; Examining Mental Health through Social Constructionism: The Language of Mental Health; An Introduction to Educational Research: Connecting Methods to Practice;* and *Digital Tools for Qualitative Research.*

Contributors

Dr Elizabeth Bromley (**MD, PhD**) is associate professor in residence in the Departments of Psychiatry and Biobehavioral Sciences and Anthropology at the University of California, Los Angeles (UCLA); and director of the DMH-UCLA Public Mental Health Partnership. Dr. Bromley completed her psychiatry residency and chief residency at Columbia University/New York State Psychiatric Institute. She is a graduate of the VA/UCLA Robert Wood Johnson Clinical Scholars program and was formerly medical director of the Greater Los Angeles VA Mental Health Intensive Case Management (MHICM) program. Her research has focused on the beliefs and concepts that underlie therapeutic practices, particularly in public mental health settings serving those diagnosed with severe mental illness. Dr. Bromley also has a research interest in physician identity and physician emotional experience, particularly as they pertain to the problem of suicide among physicians.

Dr Judy Clegg is head of division, Human Communication Sciences, Health Sciences School, University of Sheffield. Judy's research addresses the needs of children and young people with communication impairments, who grow up in high socio-economic deprivation, are involved in the criminal justice system and experience mental health difficulties from childhood to adult life. Judy is particularly interested in the complex co-morbidity between speech and language development, social disadvantage and social, emotional and mental health in children and adolescents. Judy is a Fellow of the Royal College of Speech and Language Therapists and a Trustee of ICAN, the Children's Communication Charity.

Dr Shari Couture (**PhD, R. Psych.**) is a registered psychologist with a special interest in family therapy. In addition, to her private practice she works as a sessional instructor at the University of Calgary and a clinical supervisor at the Calgary Family Therapy Centre. In her research, she uses a discursive approach to study processes and outcomes in therapy.

She has been published in a variety of journals internationally and has presented at conferences throughout North America.

Dr Sushie Dobbinson gained her PhD from University of Sheffield on repetitiveness and productivity in the conversation of adults with autism in 2000. She has worked as a lecturer in linguistics at the universities of Huddersfield, Sheffield, the Open University and York St John where she was Head of Programme from 1999–2003, when she trained as a speech and language therapist. She then worked in North East Derbyshire before moving to the Humber NHS mental health teaching Trust in 2006 where she set up the forensic SLT service in 2007. She continues to oversee the forensic service as well as being the Clinical Lead for the Humber Adult Autism Diagnosis Service.

Alison Drewett is a lecturer in speech and language therapy at De Montfort University (Leicester). She has special responsibility for the learning disability strand of the teaching and learning. She is also in her third year of a part-time PhD Studentship funded by ARC-EM, National Institute of Health Research. This is jointly supervised by Dr Michelle O'Reilly and Professor Terry Brugha at the University of Leicester. The research uses a video-reflexive ethnographic design within a critical discursive approach to investigate staff and patient interaction in mental health hospital ward rounds and focuses on collaborative care with autistic individuals. It also uses reflective interviews with staff to facilitate quality improvements in communication practices.

Gillian Eccles is an art psychotherapist who has worked in the field of mental health for a number years. She commenced her career supporting adults and then moved on to specialise in child and adolescent mental health. She currently works clinically for a children's looked after service, specialising in trauma and attachment. She is presently the psychotherapy lead for Coventry and Warwickshire NHS Partnership Trust.

Dr Mary Farrelly (PhD, MMSc, BNS, RGN, PPN) is an assistant professor of mental health and nursing in the School of Nursing, Psychotherapy, and Community Health at Dublin City University, Ireland. She has worked in clinical practice, management, and practice development in the mental health services and at national level in regulation before taking an academic post. She is a founding member of the Hearing Voices Network, Ireland, and works as a facilitator with people who hear voices.

Dr Joaquin Gaete Silva is a registered psychologist in Alberta, and works as a therapist and clinical supervisor at the Calgary Family Therapy Centre. He is a sessional instructor at Athabasca University and at the University of Calgary. He is also an adjunct researcher of the School of Psychology at Universidad Adolfo Ibáñez in Santiago, Chile. He is interested in practice, teaching, and research promoting socially just approaches to mental health, with a focus on "disruptive behaviour" in childhood and adolescence (e.g., ADHD). His research also addresses successful therapeutic processes and clinical supervision.

Dr Tania Hart is an associate professor of learning disability and mental health and head of Division for Learning Disability and Mental Health Nursing at De Montfort University. Tania has a clinical background in mental health nursing, more specifically child mental health and eating disorders. She now works in academia, whereby she is involved in mental health teaching and a number of national and international research projects focusing on adult and child well-being.

Dr Sarah Helps is a clinical psychologist and systemic psychotherapist working in the NHS and in private practice. She is trust-wide head of systemic psychotherapy at the Tavistock and Portman NHS Foundation Trust where she holds clinical, supervisory, training, and leadership roles. Her clinical practice involves working with children and young people who live out with their biological families. Recent research publications include work on the ethics of researching one's own practice, systemic practice with families where a person has an autism spectrum condition, and using autoethnography to explore use of self in relation to clinical work. Her current research interests involve the use of conversation analytic processes to explore what happens in clinical, teaching, supervision, and leadership contexts.

Dr Khalid Karim (**MMedSci, MRCPsych**) is an associate professor in medical education at University of Leicester and honorary consultant in Child and Adolescent Psychiatry at Leicestershire Partnership Trust in the United Kingdom. He has worked with children for most of his medical career and is interested in neurodevelopmental aspects of child mental health, medical education, and training of different professional groups who work with children. He has published a number of peer reviewed papers and contributed to books and other articles.

Dr Nikki Kiyimba is a senior educator and postgraduate programme lead at Bethlehem Tertiary Institute in the Bay of Plenty, New Zealand. After gaining a PhD in discursive psychology, she completed a clinical doctorate and has continued to balance a career as both a chartered clinical psychologist and an academic. She has published several books and peer reviewed journal articles, combining her knowledge as a clinical academic by engaging in research and writing in the fields of qualitative research methodology, mental health, and psychological trauma, with a focus on the application of theory to practice.

Dr Andrea LaMarre is a lecturer in critical health psychology at Massey University, New Zealand. She obtained her PhD in 2018 at the University of Guelph in the Department of Family Relations and Applied Nutrition. Her work focuses on eating disorder recovery, embodiment, gender, and health practices. She uses qualitative and arts-based approaches to explore the discursive, embodied, and affective aspects of health-related social phenomena.

Dr F. Alethea Marti (PhD, UCLA) is a linguistic anthropologist and researcher at the UCLA Center for Health Services and Society. Her research interests focus on language socialization into expertise and cultural identity among both children and adults, the role of communicative practices in building relationships and supporting shared decision-making, and the ways in which individuals make use of new technologies to both these ends. She has conducted research in Mexico and the United States on various topics including women's home businesses, adolescent gossip narratives, and adult and child mental healthcare.

Dr Elizabeth McSweeney (MRCGP) is a general practitioner in a busy inner-city primary care practice in the city of Leicester in the United Kingdom. She is involved in teaching both medical students and postgraduate trainees and is passionate about teaching clinical methods and communication skills within primary care. Her clinical interests are mental health in children and adults, neurodevelopmental presentations in primary care, and women's health and infant feeding.

Dr Andrew Reeves is an associate professor at the University of Chester. Andrew is a BACP Senior Accredited Counsellor/Psychotherapist, registered social worker, and Fellow of BACP and HEA. He has written extensively for many years on working therapeutically with people at risk of suicide, including many book chapters and several single-author texts. He has worked in a range of settings, including crisis intervention services, and supervises practitioners in schools, universities, healthcare, and independent practice. He is past-chair of BACP.

Dr Marnie Rogers-de Jong is a registered doctoral psychologist in Saskatchewan, Canada. She completed her doctor of philosophy and master of science degrees in counselling psychology at the University of Calgary. She has clinical experience providing single-session and ongoing counselling for families, couples, and individuals. Marnie currently works at a non-profit community agency and teaches counselling skills as a sessional instructor at the University of Calgary. She conducted her doctoral research at the Calgary Family Therapy Centre, where she examined interactions that facilitated a sense of "we-ness" (or mutuality and togetherness) for families in therapy using narrative and discursive methods.

Dr Inés Sametband **(PhD)** is an assistant professor with the Department of Psychology, Faculty of Arts, Mount Royal University, Canada. She is also a registered marriage and family therapist (AAMFT) and a provisionally registered psychologist in Alberta (Canada). Inés' work is informed by discursive and collaborative approaches. She is interested in how people manage cultural transitions in ways that their preferred identities are relationally recognized. Her research focuses on how cultural discourses (beliefs, explanations, values, understandings) shape therapy conversations.

Dr Olga Smoliak is an associate professor in couple therapy at the University of Guelph. She has taken a social constructionist approach to psychotherapy and has explored the links between discourse or language use and the therapeutic practices. She approaches mental illness and mental health encounters from an interactional, discursive perspective. In particular, she uses conversation analysis and discursive psychology to investigate how psychological matters are constituted discursively and how therapeutic and diagnostic interactions operate in practice.

Dr Brandon C. Yarns **(MD, MS)** is assistant professor in the University of California, Los Angeles (UCLA) Department of Psychiatry and Biobehavioral Sciences and deputy section chief for geriatric mental health at VA Greater Los Angeles Healthcare System. Dr Yarns completed a research fellowship and master's degree in research at UCLA, geriatric psychiatry fellowship at Yale University, and psychiatry residency at the University of New Mexico. He researches, teaches, and is a practitioner of intensive short-term dynamic psychotherapy and related treatments for older adults and is the author of over three dozen peer-reviewed journal articles, abstracts, and book chapters.

Dr Bonnie T. Zima **(MD MPH)** is a child psychiatrist and health services researcher. She is professor in residence in the Division of Child & Adolescent Psychiatry, associate director of the Center for Health Services & Society, and associate chair of academic affairs in the UCLA Semel Institute for Neuroscience and Human Behavior. Her research focuses on the unmet need for mental health services among high-risk child populations and the quality of child mental healthcare.

Chapter 1

Communication, mental health, and how language-based research can help in practice

Jessica Nina Lester and Michelle O'Reilly

Introduction

Communication in the field of mental health is a ubiquitous concept and one that, to some extent, has been taken for granted. However, communicating with individuals in mental health settings requires skills and training to ensure clients/patients are fully engaged in the process. Crucial to effective practice is the relationship between practitioners and their clients/patients, as well as other people involved in their care. These relationships are important at all stages of mental healthcare, including assessment, diagnosis, and treatment. Specifically, communication is important for long-term engagement, and for any required medication adherence to achieve positive outcomes.

In this chapter, we introduce the focus of the book by illuminating a body of literature that contributes significantly to the communication work in mental health. Evidence yielded from research using language-based approaches, such as discourse analytic approaches and conversation analysis, has a great deal to offer those working in practice. Such evidence has the benefit of being grounded in real-world practices due to the use of naturally occurring data, with much of this work involving or led by clinical practitioners. The focus on social inter-action and real-world practice means that the findings from such studies have the potential to make a real difference to practitioners seeking to improve their communication skills. Notably, much of the work using language-based approaches fails to reach those working in the field, due to the technical language espoused and the limited nature of many of the outlets of dissemination. Thus, in this chapter, we provide some assistance for practitioners to understand the vocabulary used, while also distilling the core messages into an appropriate and useful discourse. Furthermore, we outline the focus of the book, providing an overall synthesis of the three parts of the book and the chapters within it.

Communication and mental health

Communication is central for those working in mental health, as interacting with patients/clients, families, mental health practitioners, and representatives from other organisations and agencies is fundamental to the work. Engaging others in the consultation, especially the patient/client, is important, and the communication skills of mental health practitioners are crucial for the practice to be effective. Good communication is central for practitioners as they attempt to build a relationship with their patient/client and others involved in their care. This is necessary for longer-term engagement and rapport, but also for medication adherence, attending future appointments, and longer-term outcomes.

Despite this importance, many trainees and practitioners rely on anecdotal evidence, training courses, and experience to inform their social interactions. Often, textbooks used in courses for clinical trainees rely on experience and general approaches to communication, taking a broad approach or using models derived from experimental methods. A good example of this is psychiatry or nursing textbooks that encourage practitioners to use "open questions" without critically addressing what constitutes an open question or in what circumstances they are less effective or how such questions might be asked in a closed way (or how closed questions might be asked in an open way). Many mental health practitioners are reflexively aware of their communication skills and style, and often motivated to maintain and improve their communication competencies, especially within the modern rhetoric of evidence-based practice.

There is a substantial amount of evidence generated from communication studies, specifically from language-based approaches; studies showing the power of a single word, like that of Heritage and Robinson's (2011) work that showed the significant difference between "some" versus "any"; "Do you have any questions?" versus "Do you have some questions?" in primary care; studies showing the challenging and negative stance that why questions can take (Bolden and Robinson 2011); and studies that have highlighted the usefulness of prefacing questions with "you said x" to encourage children to talk about their problems in mental health assessments (Kiyimba and O'Reilly, 2018). This evidence is often grounded in real-world practices, and more recently, clinical authors are starting to use these approaches. Using qualitative approaches to communication, with a focus on social interaction, actual examples of communication in practice, and identifying ways in which communication works (and fails) in various circumstances, this evidence has the potential to make a real difference to the ways in which clinical practitioners work. Despite its value, and its practice-based approach to examining communication and social interaction, some of this work is written in a way that makes it inaccessible to clinical audiences. Furthermore, because of the difficult-to-access publication outlets that some of these studies appear in, much is hidden from clinical audiences, particularly those individuals who are less resourced to seek them out. However, when written in a clinically relevant and accessible way, this evidence is very useful.

Aims and objectives

Through this book, we propose that an integration of clinical experience and language-based evidence from work using approaches such as discourse and conversation analysis (although not exclusively) can provide an essential source of information for those training or working in mental health settings. Almost all chapters are led by clinical professionals with experience in using these methods, we suggest that what is offered here offers both valid and credible messages for readers. Furthermore, throughout the chapters, the complexity of the methodologies are distilled into practical and understandable messages to help practitioners who want to change or inform their practice, while simultaneously encouraging readers to go beyond the book to seek out how other work may also offer important evidence to support their daily professional lives.

Discourse and conversation analysis

Most (although not all) of the chapters draw specifically on discourse or conversation analysis to demonstrate the central role of language, the focus of social interaction, and the meaning of communication in mental health practice. While the authors of each chapter provide a short overview of their specific language-based approach in research and explain the relevant aspects of that process, we provide a brief introduction here. This description is *not* intended to be a full or detailed description of these approaches, but merely a brief introductory overview.

Discourse analysis

Discourse analysis is an umbrella term that refers to a range of approaches that examine the use of language in social interaction. Discourse analysis spans several disciplines and there is variability in how discourse is conceptualised and analysed (Georgaca, 2014). However, all discourse approaches focus on language and meaning in talk and text. That is, there is agreement across the various approaches to discourse analysis that language is central to the meanings of the human world (Spong, 2010) and that it is through language that social life is performed.

There are different theoretical strands of discourse analysis. Those that focus on the macro-processes of social interaction and those that focus on the micro-processes of social interaction is a common distinction that has been made. Those that focus on the macro-processes include approaches like critical discourse analysis, critical discursive psychology, and Foucauldian discourse analysis (see Wooffitt, 2005 for an overview). These macro-focused discourse approaches examine the socially available discourses that people draw upon when presenting their views and experiences and tend to be concerned with power, social domination, and inequality (Georgaca, 2014). These types of discourse analysis are concerned with the role of discourse in the production of power within certain social structures to see how discourses might sustain and legitimise social inequality (Wooffitt, 2005). In so doing, these discourse analysts take an explicit socio-political position and focus on the production of the dominance of elite groups or organisations and consider how these are reproduced by the talk or text (van Dijk, 2008). Those discourse analysis types that focus on micro-processes of social interaction include approaches like discursive psychology (Edwards and Potter 1992). This type of discourse approach tends to have a closer alignment with conversation analysis and focuses more on how meaning is co-created between interlocutors. These discourse analysts prefer to collect data that represents real-world interactions and argue that any speech act can only be analysed in a meaningful way by reference to the situated nature of the talk (Edwards and Potter, 1992).

Conversation analysis

Conversation analysis, as a distinct qualitative methodology, is designed to examine language in interaction in terms of how the turns of talk are designed to perform certain social actions (Antaki, 2011). To put it simply, conversation analysts study social interactions, attending to the ordered and patterned nature of the talk itself. Indeed, those practicing conversation analysis study "talk-in-interaction" (Drew and Heritage, 1992). Although conversation analysis is interested in language, the main object of its study is the interactional organisation of social activities; that is, the production of talk and sense obtained through a sequential structure in terms of the practical social accomplishment (Hutchby and Wooffitt, 2008). To achieve its analytical goals, conversation analysts collect data from the real world, referred to as naturally occurring data. Naturally occurring data are those recordings (or natural texts) of actual practices, such as classroom interactions, therapy conversations, or police-witness interviews (see Kiyimba, Lester, and O'Reilly, 2019). In so doing, conversation analysts focus on what people actually say and do, rather than what they report they say and do (McCabe, 2006).

More recently, conversation analysts have turned significant attention to talk and interaction within institutional settings, and more scholars have begun to consider the value and application of their findings to practitioners. Therefore, a distinction has been drawn between basic and applied conversation analysis (Antaki, 2011). Basic (sometimes referred to as pure) conversation analysis examines mundane and commonplace interactions (McCabe, 2006), whereas applied conversation analysis tends to (although not exclusively) focus on interactions within institutional settings (Lester and O'Reilly, 2019). Notably, the application of conversation analysis to institutional talk is not necessarily related to solving problems of institutions, but instead focuses on how those institutions carry out their institutional business successfully (Antaki, 2011; O'Reilly et al., 2020).

Relevance of discourse and conversation analysis to mental health

We argue that language-based approaches are useful approaches to examine mental health. This is because mental states and psychiatric categories are produced through and within language (Harper, 1995), as the very idea of "normality" or "sanity", "pathology", and "insanity" are typifications that start with observation and social interaction (Roca-Cuberes, 2008). The focus on language therefore has worked to reframe conceptualisations of mental health and mental ill health, as well as its management, shifting the emphasis away from biomedical explanations to interpersonal and social-cultural ones (Georgaca, 2014).

Importantly, discourse and conversation analytic approaches are also important in understanding the institutional business related to mental health. For example, by using these approaches new perspectives have been brought to the fore on therapy, counselling, and psychiatric care. This is especially useful as a focus on language for analysis is congruent with therapeutic practice as both take place through language and focus on meaning-making (McLeod, 2001). Notably, this is not to say that these approaches tell practitioners how to conduct therapy effectively; rather, they highlight how clients and therapists create the therapeutic process together (Streeck, 2010). In other words, these approaches provide evidence that is tangible, empirical, and useful for examining the process of therapeutic change (Strong, Busch, and Couture, 2008; Tseliou et al., in press).

A note about transcription

Throughout the chapters, it is the case that most of the authors represent the extracts of data through a transcript of the talk. In so doing, many of them use the traditional transcription conventions of Gail Jefferson (see Jefferson, 2004). There are, of course, debates about the role of transcription in re-search but typically it is seen as an active process (Lapadat, 2000), and in many language-based approaches there is a motivation to reflect not just *what* was said but also *how* it was said. The Jefferson system allows analysts to represent the talk in this way through a complex series of symbols to represent the different ways that people talk, capturing emphasis, para-linguistic features, pauses, and so on (Hepburn and Bolden, 2017). For those practicing conversation analysis, transcription is also a core *analytic* activity as the analyst engages with the data and develops a deeper understanding of the communication process (Roberts and Robinson, 2004).

The Jefferson system utilised by many practicing discourse and con-versation analysts pays particular attention to detail. Notably, in the process of transcription, there is no correction of grammar or pronunciation (Hepburn and Bolden, 2017). The complexity of the system, however, is one that has to be learned and can feel very unfamiliar and challenging for those

Table 1.1 Jefferson transcription symbols (Jefferson, 2004)

Symbol	Description
(.)	A full stop (period) inside brackets denotes a micro-pause, a notable pause but of no significant length.
(0.2)	A number inside brackets denotes a timed pause. This is a pause long enough to time and subsequently show in transcription.
[ ]	Square brackets denote a point where overlapping speech occurs and ends.
>speech<	Arrows surrounding talk like these show that the pace of the speech has quickened.
<speech>	Arrows in this direction show that the pace of the speech has slowed down.
Underlined	When a word or part of a word is underlined, it denotes a raise in volume or emphasis.
↑	When an upward arrow appears, it means there is a rise in intonation.
↓	When a downward arrow appears, it means there is a lowering of intonation.
→	An arrow like this denotes a sentence of interest to the analyst.
CAPITALS	Where capital letters appear, it denotes that something was said loudly or even shouted.
:::	Colons appear to represent elongated speech, a stretched sound.

who have not seen it before. Therefore, we encourage you to engage with the basic symbols before you try to read the extracts of data in the book. Please see Table 1.1 for an overview of the most common symbols.

The structure of the book

In total, this book comprises 14 chapters (including this one). The book is usefully divided into three broad parts to reflect the conceptual areas of research and their foci. In Part One, we focus on research with children and families, presenting research studies that consider helpful ways to communicate with younger clients/patients. In Part Two, the focus moves to adults, whereby research studies that have explored communication with adults with mental health need are reported. In Part Three, the final part of the book, the focus shifts slightly, as we reflect on the learning journeys of clinical practitioners who have undertaken research, reflecting on the process of conducting the project and offering lessons learned in the quest for evidence.

Part One of the book

The chapters in the first part of the book, which focus on children, young people, and families, covers a range of areas in mental health practice and settings. This reflects the expertise of a range of practitioners creating a cross-disciplinary approach to understanding communication with younger populations in multi-party interactions. Mental health work with children and young people frequently also involves parents (or primary carers) and other family members. Although this is not always the case, it is often necessary for practitioners to communicate with children and young people while their parents listen, contribute, interrupt or interject. Part One, therefore, provides an entire tool kit for those who work with children and young people to consider how to engage this population, build rapport, assess risk, and encourage disclosure.

The chapters in this part of the book examine a range of different settings of mental health practice and we list here the abstracts from the chapters in Part One, starting with chapter two.

Chapter 2, by Karim, McSweeney, and O'Reilly: Communication with children is central to child mental health settings. In the UK, children are referred to Child and Adolescent Mental Health Services (CAMHS), usually by the general practitioner. The first step for CAMHS is to determine if the child has a diagnosable condition which is examined through an initial assessment. Utilising video-recorded naturally occurring data from 28 families attending their first appointment at CAMHS, we focus on the strategies that are empirically shown to be effective in engaging children in conversation. In the chapter we highlight important and useful practical communication strategies for multidisciplinary mental health teams who assess children for mental health difficulties. We focus our key messages round a range of identified techniques looking at how practitioners ask questions and the implications of this for engagement. Specifically, we examine the nature and frequency of questions, including exploring the child's perceived reasons for attendance.

Key words: child mental health; communication; question design; qualitative

Chapter 3, by Smoliak et al.: Family therapists often work with more than one family member in the room. Involving multiple family members in therapy can help avoid the pathologizing of one family member and also help address clients' relational concerns more effectively. However, working with multiple family members simultaneously is not without challenges and may give rise to practical dilemmas (e.g., how to join with and validate one client's account without jeopardizing the alliance with other family members). In this chapter, we identify three practical questions or dilemmas family therapists may encounter in their practice and argue that discourse analytic (discursive) research focused on language use in social interaction can help therapists recognize and navigate these dilemmas. Discursive methods of inquiry can help therapists recognize how they already practice in collaborative, non-blaming, and neutral ways and help further enhance the collaborative potential of their practice.

Key words: family therapy; discourse; communication; discursive inquiry; practice-based evidence

Chapter 4, by Kiyimba: *The chapter focuses on one specific aspect of communicating with children and young people, which is in relation to the use of reflected speech. Reflected speech re-introduces a previously discussed topic into the current conversational interaction, but rather than reporting on what someone else has said, the speaker reflects the words of the addressee. In effect, rather than using the canonical "he said/she said", the speaker would use the preface "you said". This preface will be shown to be part of a sequence of interactional turns established between the two speakers wherein the topic embedded in the reflected speech is established as an accepted basis for proceeding. In a clinical setting, using this either as part of the assessment or the therapy stage, can assist the therapeutic process between adult therapist and the young clients that they are working with, by enabling shared access to which topics of conversation are made immediately relevant. As a clinical psychologist, the practical applications of using this strategy are explored and the key arguments reiterated.*

Key words: communication; child mental health; you-said questions; qualitative; assessments

Chapter 5, by Clegg: *Research supports an association between children's communication needs and their social, emotional, and mental health (SEMH). Vulnerable populations of children and adolescents have a higher-than-expected prevalence of communication needs. Importantly, these communication needs are not consistently identified nor addressed. In response to this, the profession of speech and language therapy advocates the involvement of speech and language therapists in health, education, and social services to accurately assess the communication needs of these children and young people and to provide evidence-based interventions to facilitate more effective communication between the child, their family, and professionals. This chapter discusses the research identifying the communication needs of these vulnerable children and young people. The role of the speech and language therapist is explained and specific approaches that all professionals can adopt to enable effective communication advocated. Case examples of children will be used to illustrate the profiles of communication needs and how communication interventions can address these.*

Key words: speech and language therapy; communication; children; vulnerability

Chapter 6, by Kiyimba, Karim, and O'Reilly: *In the UK, Child and Adolescent Mental Health Services (CAMHS) provide a service for children and families to assess, diagnose, and treat children and young people with emotional, behavioural, and neurodevelopmental conditions. In child mental health, it is* *usual for mental health practitioners to assess risk to ascertain whether the child self-harms or has any suicidal intent. However, communicating with children and young people about risk is a delicate and somewhat challenging endeavour for practitioners. We suggest that this may in part be due to the complexity of communicating with children about this sensitive topic. For the chapter, we draw upon 28 video-recorded initial mental health assessments with children aged 6–17 years old. By using conversation analysis, we identify practices that engaged children effectively and provided space for children to elaborate on the risks when an affirmative response was provided, but not feel uneasy when the question was disconfirmed. In concluding our chapter, we demonstrate for those working in clinical practice best practices and provide advice regarding how to ask children and young people about their feelings, intentions, and behaviours.*

Key words: self-harm; suicide; children; risk; conversation analysis

Chapter 7, by Marti and Zima*: Parent engagement is crucial to the success of paediatric medication treatment: After leaving the clinic, the parent is the one in charge of administering the medication, monitoring symptoms and side effects, and making in-the-moment decisions if problems arise. Child ADHD treatment is complicated by the fact that new medications must be titrated – gradually increasing a dose over several weeks while carefully monitoring the child's reactions – so parents become skilled in basic medication safety monitoring. Successful treatment depends on good communication and mutual trust between parent and physician, as well as the creation of a non-judgmental space where parents' concerns and fears can be addressed. In this chapter we examine strategies that U.S. child psychiatrists at a community mental health clinic use to build such partnerships. Data are drawn from video-recordings of early-stage clinic appointments collected for a pilot test of a mobile web application for paediatric ADHD medication management. We illustrate how both psychiatrists and parents draw on multiple resources (including visual charts and verbal descriptions) and use strategies ranging from inclusive language to the construction of hypothetical future scenarios, and we provide tips for practitioners to implement with their own clients.*

Key words: ADHD; medication management; technology; conversation analysis; parent-provider shared decision-making; child mental health

Part Two of the book

The chapters in the second part of the book, which focus on adults, also cover a range of areas in mental health practice and settings. This part of the book reflects the expertise of different practitioners exploring communication with adult clients/patients from different disciplinary perspectives. Mental health work with adults reflects a spectrum of different mental health needs and conditions and practitioners navigate various challenges in this communication. Part Two, therefore, provides an entire tool kit for those who practice with adults in mental health, to consider how to engage this population, build rapport, assessment of risk, and encourage disclosure. As such, Part Two of the book synthesises contemporary research that utilises language-based approaches for the study of adult mental health, while highlighting the practical implications of these core messages.

Chapter 8, by Dobbinson: Pseudologia fantastica (PF), also known as pathological lying or mythomania, involves the production of extravagant or incredible tales which have no obvious motive for gain or advantage. When PF occurs in the context of a forensic setting, clinicians often interpret it as a barrier to therapy, as purposefully rejecting of the engagement or even of the co-interactant personally. Instances of PF encountered on a forensic learning disability ward, selected to be typical of the individuals and the setting, in this chapter are examined as they occur spontaneously within the talk of individual patients conversing with clinical staff. The moment by moment construction of PF by participants is analysed using CA and DA and situated in terms of the forensic context in which the interaction takes place, as well as the wider context of the patients' lives and experiences. Interestingly, recipients often appear to collaborate in the production of PF as well as clearly marking recognition of the PF turns as deception. The analysis suggests that PF is an emergent product of interaction rather than an individual choice about behaviour.

Key words: mental health; pseudologia fantastica; forensic setting; conversation analysis

Chapter 9, by Yarns and Bromley: Understanding our patients' feelings is critical to providing high-quality mental healthcare. Yet, patients seeking mental healthcare often have difficulty reporting their feelings in response to direct questions in a clinical interview. Using interview data from Partners in Care, a randomized-controlled trial of quality improvement for depression, we provide examples of the complex and often baffling responses chronically depressed older patients may use when directly asked to report their feelings, and, in an effort to make sense of these responses, we delineate three qualitatively different categories of words patients use to describe their feelings – specific feeling words, vague feeling words, and physical words. We describe in detail the theoretical and empirical justification for these categories and explain how listening for patterns of words that patients use to describe their emotional experiences can augment the standard clinical interview and self-report checklists to improve communication about patients' feelings. We then demonstrate how eliciting specific feeling words provides more actionable information for the mental health clinician than vague or physical words and review particularly effective techniques clinicians can use to elicit specific feeling words, such as repeating questions and encouraging specificity and detail.

Key words: depression; mental health; feelings; communication

Chapter 10, by Farrelly: *This chapter considers issues of communication in mental health nursing through an exploration of the use of language. Farrelly draws on her own research that considered the discursive construction of mental health problems in print media using Foucauldian discourse analytic methodology. The use of psychiatrically oriented language and pessimistic talk is discussed. Strategies for development of communication patterns that allow the person's voice to be foregrounded and language congruent with a philosophy of recovery emphasising personal strengths rather than weakness are considered. Examples from practice scenarios are provided as a basis for reflection.*

Key words: discourse analysis; mental health nursing; language; communication

Chapter 11, by Reeves: *The purpose of this chapter is to consider the importance of discourse-based approaches in working with people who present at suicide risk, particularly in the context of a tools-based, risk-factor informed culture in mental health. Current mental health practice is generally informed by a risk-factor approach to working with suicide, where the task of the mental health worker is to ascertain risk factors to help predict likelihood of a suicide attempt. While tools and questionnaires can inform some understanding of suicide potential, research suggests they are typically a blunt instrument in helping the practitioner – and suicidal person – to fully understand the complexity and multi-layered phenomenological process of suicide. The chapter will argue that while such tools provide important contextual meaning, it is only in a dialogic engagement that a more purposeful exploration of suicidality, which enhances understanding for both the practitioner and suicidal individual, can be achieved. The chapter concludes with some evidence-informed, accessible, good-practice guidelines to contribute to the development of knowledge and practice in discourse-based approaches to working with suicide risk.*

Key words: suicide; mental health; risk; discourse; communication

Part Three of the book

The chapters in the third part of the book have a different emphasis, as they move away from practice in clinical contexts, examining the value and process of doing mental health research and supervision. In this part of the book, practitioners working in the field of mental health examine and consider the relevance and importance of undertaking communication research in mental health and the value of clinical supervision. In so doing they reflect their dual role of researcher (or supervisor) and practitioner, while contemplating the type of evidence and knowledge produced. Part Three of the book therefore provides not only discussion about communication and tools for best practice, but also discussion about how to do this kind of research and its value from a practice-based perspective.

Chapter 12, by Drewett: Speech and language therapists work across different settings with a varied client group from children to adults and in healthcare, education, and social care. Much of this work is embedded with a social model of disability so that the focus of SALT recommendations and training is often aimed at communication partners rather than changes by the individual client. Drewett's PhD study is focused on adults with autism who are admitted into generic mental settings, with a specific interest in their experiences of decision-making regarding their care and discharge in team meetings. The focus of this chapter is on the potential value of a CA approach for SALTs. CA views communication as produced in the sequence of turn-taking in interactions so the locus of responsibility for what evolves out of interaction is seen in the interaction partners and not just the individual. It is suggested that these approaches can contribute to this area of clinical work. CA can identify where there is a communication difficulty and how and when that difficulty emerges.

Key words: speech and language therapy; communication; mental health; autism; learning disabilities

Chapter 13, by Helps: Supervision plays a vital role in the delivery of safe, effective, reflective clinical practice. Supervision of work with families is multi-layered and includes both detailed scrutiny of how family members communicate with each other as well as exploration of how therapists build effective communication with those in the family system. Retrospective supervision based on the clinicians' memory and clinical notes is the most common type of supervision once a clinician is qualified. However, this supervisory form often lacks the detail and depth compared with review of what actually happened within a clinical session based on review of a recording. This chapter focusses on the benefits of using conversation analytic tools within supervision to explore and ultimately improve therapist-family communication. Based on a review of literature and a detailed practice-example, Helps *shows the benefits of starting supervisory conversations with conversation-analytic examination of video-tape of communication* and *shows how words and embodied actions can tell different stories about the process of communication and so need to be considered together. Micro-practices of spoken and embodied communication are connected to issues of power and social diversity. Overall, it is concluded that the costs of making and carefully examining recordings of clinical work within supervision are outweighed by the learning gained.*

Key words: conversation analysis; supervision; reflective clinical practice; communication; family interaction

Chapter 14, by Hart and Eccles: Mental health nurse and associate professor, Tania Hart, and colleague, Gillian Eccles, who is a lead art psychotherapist, reflect on their learning journey undertaking mental health research, audit, and service evaluations with children and adolescents diagnosed with emotional and behavioural conditions. Good interpersonal skills and communication is essential for effective engagement with young participants, as this maximises the robustness and value of the research data produced. This chapter explores the benefits and challenges of doing this kind of work, whilst discussing the necessity of focusing on the differing engagement, communication, and language styles to promote effective child-focussed enquiry which then has the potential to benefit clinical practice.

Key words: communication; research; young people; engagement; child-centred

Intended audience and conclusion

Communication skills are central for mental health practitioners and this book provides an evidence base for what works well in communicating with patients/clients and shows why and how it works well. This book is likely to appeal to a broad international audience, and is accessible for a wide range of professionals, students/clinical trainees, and academics from a range of disciplines involving mental health. This book is useful for psychiatrists, psychologists, nurses, family therapists, speech and language therapists, play therapists, cognitive behaviour therapists, occupational therapists, psychotherapists, art therapists, child counsellors, social workers, social policy developers, and voluntary workers. It may be of use to youth workers, SENCOs, classroom assistants, and teachers if they have an interest in mental health. This book is a valuable resource for undergraduate and postgraduate students in psychology and medicine (potentially also sociology). We believe that this book is especially useful for trainees on specialised counselling and therapy courses, the clinical psychology doctorate, and other forms of mental health training. The book may also be useful for academics interested in mental health and managers in mental health services. Notably, another potential audience is graduate students and postgraduate students enrolled in graduate-level qualitative courses, as well as more specialized courses in conversation analysis and discourse analysis.

References

Antaki, C., 2011. Six kinds of applied conversation analysis. In: Antaki, C. (Ed.), *Applied Conversation Analysis: intervention and Change in Institutional Talk*. Palgrave MacMillan, Hampshire, pp. 1–14.

Bolden, G., Robinson, J., 2011. Soliciting accounts with why-interrogatives in conversation. *J. Commun. 61*, 94–119.

Drew, P., Heritage, J., 1992. Analyzing talk at work: an introduction. In: Drew, D. and Heritage, J. (Eds.), *Talkat Work: Interaction in Institutional Settings*. Cambridge University Press, Cambridge, pp. 3–65.

Georgaca, E., 2014. Discourse analytic research on mental distress: A critical overview. *J. Ment. Health 23* (2), 55–61.

Edwards, D., Potter, J., 1992. *Discursive Psychology*. SAGE, London.

Harper, D., 1995. Discourse analysis and 'mental health'. *J. Ment. Health 4*, 347–357.

Hepburn, A., Bolden, G., 2017. *Transcribing for Social Research*. SAGE, London.

Heritage, J., Robinson, J., 2011. 'Some' versus 'any' medical issues: encouraging patients to reveal their unmet concerns. In: Antaki, C. (Ed.), *Applied Conversation Analysis: Intervention and Change in Institutional Talk*. Palgrave MacMillan, Hampshire, pp. 15–31.

Hutchby, I., Wooffitt, R., 2008. *Conversation Analysis*, third ed. Polity Press, Cambridge.

Jefferson, G., 2004. Glossary of transcript symbols with an introduction. In: Lerner, G.H. (Ed.), *Conversation Analysis: Studies from the First Generation*. John Benjamins, Amsterdam, pp. 13–31.

Kiyimba, N., Lester, J., O'Reilly, M. 2019. *Using Naturally Occurring Data in Health Research: A Practical Guide*. Springer, Germany.

Kiyimba, N., O'Reilly, M., 2018. Reflecting on what 'you said' as a way of re-introducing difficult topics in child mental health assessments. *Child. Adolesc. Ment. Health 23* (3), 148–154.

Lapadat, J., 2000. Problematizing transcription: purpose, paradigm and quality. *Int. J. Soc. Res. Methodol. 3* (3), 203–219.

Lester, J., O'Reilly, M., 2019. *Applied Conversation Analysis: Social Interaction in Institutional Settings*. SAGE, Thousand Oaks, CA.

McCabe, R., 2006. Conversation analysis. In: Slade, M., Priebe, S. (Eds.), *Choosing Methods in Mental Health Research: Mental Health Research from Theory to Practice*. Routledge, Hove, pp. 24–46.

McLeod, J., 2001. *Qualitative Research in Counseling and Psychotherapy*. SAGE, London.

O'Reilly, M., Kiyimba, N., Lester, J., Muskett, T., 2020. Reflective Interventionist Conversation Analysis. *Discourse & Communication 14* (6), 619–634.

Roberts, F., Robinson, J., 2004. Interobserver agreement on first-stage conversation analytic transcription. *Health Commun. Res. 30* (3), 376–410.

Roca-Cuberes, C., 2008. Membership categorisation and professional insanity ascription. *Discourse Stud. 10* (4), 543–570.

Spong, S., 2010. Discourse analysis: rich pickings for counsellors and therapists. *Counselling Psychotherapy Res. 10* (1), 67–74.

Streeck, U., 2010. A psychotherapist's view of conversation analysis. In: Peräkylä, A., Antaki, C., Vehvilainen, S., Leudar, I. (Eds.), *Conversation Analysis and Psychotherapy*. Cambridge University Press, Cambridge, pp. 173–187.

Strong, T., Busch, R., Couture, S., 2008. Conversational evidence in therapeutic dialogue. *J. Marital. Family Ther. 34* (3), 388–405.

Tseliou, E., Burck, C., Forbat, E., Strong, T., O'Reilly, M., in press. The discursive performance of change process in systemic and constructionist therapies: a systematic meta-synthesis review of in-session therapy discourse. *Family Process*.

van Dijk, T., 2008. *Discourse and Power*. Palgrave, Hampshire.

Wooffitt, R., 2005. *Conversation Analysis and Discourse Analysis: A Comparative and Critical Introduction*. SAGE, London.

Part I

Communication with children and families

Chapter 2

Communication in child mental health

Improving engagement with families

Khalid Karim, Elizabeth McSweeney, and Michelle O'Reilly

Introduction

> *"The good physician treats the disease; the great physician treats the patient who has the disease."*
>
> Sir William Osler (1849–1919)

Communication, from the Latin verb *communicare* meaning "to share", is the ability to transfer information from one person to another. We communicate all the time in a variety of formats which have become increasingly complex in the modern world. However, the use of speech and other forms of personal communication remain the most common and often, most powerful. While in contemporary practice there is a growing focus on social media, messaging, and the use of mobile technology, it is still the use of the spoken word that dominates. The way in which we speak with others is often taken for granted but remains a hugely influential way of gathering information from others and for expressing our own thoughts and feelings. In other words, social interaction is crucial for society to function.

At its simplest, communication requires a sender, a recipient, and a message. What is often not appreciated, though, is that this is a highly complex process that can be affected by a huge range of factors and misinterpreting others can be deceptively easy. The integration of verbal and non-verbal communication helps to reinforce and strengthen our message, builds rapport, or creates trust or shows that we are listening.

In healthcare settings, communication is a central aspect of any encounter. The practitioner must be able to communicate with their client/patient effectively for the encounter to serve its function. As noted, communication is not as straightforward and simple as it may ostensibly seem. This is exacerbated further in situations where the practitioner is communicating with multiple parties, especially if one or more members are children or adolescents. Communicating with children/young people and families requires additional skills, reflection, and training. In this chapter, therefore, we focus on this specifically by providing some core messages that we have learned from our own research. We turn our attention to specific communication practices that may facilitate the engagement of children or young people in mental health settings and provide recommendations for ways to communicate effectively with families. We therefore begin the chapter by critically considering the value of communication in healthcare interactions and move our focus more specifically toward the challenges of communicating with children and families.

"Just listen to the patient, he/she is telling you the diagnosis"

Communication in the healthcare environment remains one of the most important but often overlooked means to provide good quality of care. William Osler, the 19th-century Canadian physician and often regarded as the "Father of Modern Medicine" recognised the importance of allowing patients to tell their story (see Centor, 2007). Patients are key players in healthcare and should be recognised as experts in their own health as it is necessary to understand their perspective. Despite increasing reliance on sophisticated technologies and innovative diagnostic tools and treatments, it is the one-to-one interaction that is crucial to all aspects of care. Good communication allows the patient to provide their perspective, enables the practitioner to ask the right questions, come to the correct conclusion, and communicate this information effectively. Michael Balint (1957), an influential psychoanalyst, in *The Doctor, His Patient and the Illness,* talked about the therapeutic impact of the doctor themselves on the patient – the "doctor as the drug" – and how this could only be achieved through advanced communication and engagement skills leading to a therapeutic relationship.

There is no universally accepted definition of engagement but put simply, it is involving people in their own care with patients and practitioners working together to improve health. When successful, it can build rapport and enhance relationships, improve motivation, and the subsequent outcomes of treatment. In addition to the obvious benefits to the patient it is cost effective and generates increased levels of satisfaction for the practitioner. Numerous factors influence engagement and while it is not always easy to translate into everyday practice, engagement needs to remain paramount in healthcare interactions. We list some of the reasons why engaging children in their healthcare is so important in Box 2.1.

Engaging with children and young people

Engagement is an essential aspect of working with families. Children, however, should not be considered mini-adults and communicating with children and young people has its own challenges. Reasons such as chronological age, intellectual and linguistic ability, or emotional development as

---

Box 2.1   The importance of engagement in healthcare

Why engagement through effective communication is important

Effective communication is a cornerstone of clinical practice and there are many reasons for this, and these include:

* Improves trust
* Reduces anxiety
* Makes everyone feel included
* Increases clinician satisfaction
* Helps with decision making and diagnostic thinking
* Improves adherence to treatment
* Improves patient outcomes
* Improves attendance at appointments
* Reduces complaints

---

well as the presence of other adults affect this interaction; cultural and social factors also play a role. It has been established that involving children and young people in their healthcare leads to better outcomes (Chu and Kendall, 2004; Lewis et al., 1984) but evidence suggests that this does not always happen and they are often relegated to a minor role, with their views sidelined (Day et al., 2011; Persson et al., 2017). The addition of a third party such as a parent (or legal guardian) affects the interpersonal dynamic, adding complexity and has been termed a "triadic consultation" (Cahill and Papageorgiou, 2007). As parents and other family members can present with feelings of distress or frustration and tend to be vocal about these, the needs of the parent may take priority, leaving children or young people feeling that their views are not taken seriously (Buston, 2002), but children's voices are important. Despite it being shown that children and young people account for up to one-third of primary care consultations, they often have little meaningful involvement and the conversation predominately centres between the adult and the doctor (Cahill and Papageorgiou, 2007).

Nonetheless, in a contemporary society children and young people are voicing concerns about wanting to have a say in the decisions made about them and the United Nations Convention on the Rights of the Child (1989) underpins this position. This global treaty has been highly influential on healthcare practices, particularly in the UK, and has driven an agenda of child-centred practice. However, there is no clear consensus on what constitutes child-centred practice, and this makes it challenging to implement in the real world of healthcare. Most practitioners consider themselves child-centred in the sense that they believe they listen to children and respect their views, but this may not be reflected in their actual practice where there are many competing demands. Training on communicating and engaging with children may be variable across professional groups and tends to be learnt through observing others and experience over time. In the field of mental health this is especially important, as listening to children and making sense of their experiences is central to assessing, diagnosing, and treating any mental health need. Furthermore, in the process of recognising that mental health need may exist, there is a pre-developed pathway of help-seeking by the family and communicating the challenges faced is important in understanding the nature of the presenting problem and assessing any risk (see Kiyimba, Karim, and O'Reilly, this volume).

Child mental health

Globally, the number of children experiencing mental health conditions has increased dramatically over the last few years (Bor et al., 2014). There has been a significant increase in all areas of mental health conditions, particularly in the diagnosis of neurodevelopmental conditions such as autism or attention deficit hyperactivity disorder (NHS Digital, 2018). The number of children who self-harm and have eating disorders has also risen and this has caused considerable concern for healthcare, governments, and society (NHS Digital, 2018). While some aspects of the rise in prevalence could be due to increased recognition of these difficulties as there have been instrumental attempts to raise awareness about mental health generally, there does appear to be an actual increase of these conditions, with the causes unclear. This is likely due to the multi-factorial profile of any mental health condition (Dogra et al., 2017).

Child mental health conditions can arise from diverse and interconnected factors, which have a biological or genetic, psychological, and social basis. For example, children are especially sensitive to the effects of poverty and parental mental health, and factors like poor sleep and peer relationships can have a profound impact on them. The acknowledgement that many adult mental health problems have their origin in childhood highlights the need for practitioners to engage well with children and their families to achieve better long-term outcomes.

Child mental health assessments

Child mental health conditions present in a wide range of settings from primary care, education, social care, policing, and the voluntary sector. The average primary care consultation in the UK is for only 10 minutes and during this time the family put forward their concerns about the child or young person. Notably, only a small percentage of these children have needs specific or severe enough to be seen in secondary care. However, when there is suspected strong mental health need, and primary care physicians (like the general practitioner [GP]) feel that there is a case, they may refer to a specialist mental health service. In the UK, these are called Child and Adolescent Mental Health Services (CAMHS). The referral thus requests that an initial mental health assessment is conducted to determine if there is specific mental health need. In other words, this is an initial screening appointment to identify symptoms, ascertain risk, and provide an initial formulation of what the presenting problem may be (Mash and Hunsley, 2005). The purpose and outcomes of these assessments are diverse, and the interactions may vary in length (O'Reilly et al., 2015). Clearly, involving and engaging children in all settings, primary or secondary care, is important to accomplishing the best outcome and to ensure that any referral onward (either to specialist services or for diagnosis and treatment) is warranted.

There is no consistent model or way of assessing children in a specialist secondary care environment. Most children or young people are seen as an outpatient, although depending on the problem and type of service they can also been seen in their home or at school. Generally, the child or young person and their family meet with either one or two practitioners to explore the story behind the referral. They may be seen alone to gain their perspective for part or most of the assessment. Additionally, practitioners can seek information from third-party sources such as family or any other agencies involved. A formulation and management plan are generated at the end of this process and a decision regarding if there is or is not mental health need is made. The first assessment can be of significant therapeutic value with the all parties benefiting from just being listened to.

Research into communication with children

Despite the significant increase in research over the past few years, there remains limited published research focusing on real-world empirical evidence of communication with children and young people, particularly generated from clinical settings. There has been more research into communication with adults, particularly in general practice and much of the literature looks at the doctor–patient relationship. In younger populations the research arises mostly from paediatric outpatient settings, but also again mostly from primary care and predominantly in relation to physical health. Ultimately therefore, there is much less evidence for practitioners to utilise in relation to interacting with children and young people in mental health settings, and even less in relation to first assessments.

There is a body of work that has examined communication with families in the context of treatment for mental health need (see Marti and Zima, this volume, for an example of communication with parents). For example, family therapy does have a significant body of work (see Tseliou et al., 2020, for a review). This is useful and some of the core messages are certainly translatable to other settings. For example, this literature illustrates how central the family *system* is to the behaviour and emotional state of its members and encourages families to work together in a holistic way to promote functioning (Dallos and Draper, 2010; Smoliak et al., this volume). Communication work in family therapy has pointed to the importance of therapeutic alliance for change process to be successful showing that communication between therapist and family members is crucial (Strong, Busch, and Couture, 2008), and other work has highlighted how important the engagement of the child is for treatment (O'Reilly and Parker, 2013). Other research that is translatable in the context of mental health communication has been generated in the field of child counselling (see Hutchby, 2002; 2010) and in paediatric consultations (Stivers, 2002). For example, Hutchby illustrated the central role of "active listening" to encourage participation of children in the encounter and highlighted the powerful position children can occupy when making claims to insufficient knowledge (e.g., "I don't know") to resist providing answers to questions. Likewise, Stivers noted the relevance and challenge of engaging children in healthcare interactions, illustrating through a conversational coding strategy that children occupied very little of the conversation in terms of minutes of the appointment (Stivers, 2002).

The lessons learned and messages presented are, however, very much in the context of families undergoing *treatment* in the form of *therapy* or *counselling,* rather than in the context of the first assessment which has a different goal, a different function, and a different agenda. While the important recommendations and messages for practitioners can be taken from this evidence base representing different settings, the body of work is small compared to those that rely on questionnaires, randomised controlled trials, and other forms of measurement, and yet, it is these kinds of communication studies that shine a light on real-world practices that are arguably the most enlightening and realistic. They do not rely on artificial situations or retrospective accounts from practitioners, but instead focus on *what* practitioners are doing, and *how* they are doing it. It is therefore necessary to examine how communication unfolds and how practice is accomplished in real-world mental health settings, especially in the context of the initial mental health assessment, as this sets up the trajectory for the child or young person and their family and directs whether and what type of support or services they might subsequently receive.

We recognise however that these person-centred, practice-based evidence types of research are challenging to undertake and difficult to acquire funds for. In a competitive research environment, funding in child mental health research is especially difficult to secure. Research into communication can be difficult to execute and lack clear outcomes, especially the favoured measurable outcomes. So, you may be wondering why we bother. There are so many important reasons: it informs contemporary practice as communication is at the heart of all that practitioners in mental health do; it is fundamental for training as practitioners learn how to engage children and young people in any consultation; and involving children or young people in research ensures that children's voices help shape future services and improve quality of care. This is crucial to promote a child-centred healthcare service in any country, to adhere to the UN convention of children's rights, but most importantly of all, to improve quality of care and outcomes, essential in the modern quality improvement agenda in the field.

Our research

We ourselves view communication and child-centred practice as at the heart of any mental health practice. The aim of our research project was therefore to investigate the real-world interactions between families and practitioners during initial mental health assessments to explore the communication practices, with a goal of highlighting good practice and where needed, improving care. The study was conducted in one CAMH service in the UK. We completed a rigorous NHS ethics process to ensure we complied with all ethical governance procedures. We subsequently collected a sample of all consenting first appointments but excluded urgent and acute referrals because of the likelihood of distress. In practice this meant that all members of the interaction, adult/child, clinical/lay provided consent (or assent) at the beginning of the recording and again at the end to provide space for withdrawal post-event. In this setting, the assessments were conducted by an outpatient multi-disciplinary team which included consultant, staff grade, and trainee psychiatrists, clinical and assistant psychologists, community psychiatric nurses, psychotherapists, and occupational therapists. In total, our study included all 29 of the staff from that team.

Our study included 28 families who consented to be video-recorded for our study and this provided 2240 minutes of data, as the average assessment was 90 minutes long. Mostly assessments were conducted by two professionals, although some had a third person observing or a medical/nursing student in attendance. The children and young people ranged from 6–17 years old, with a mean age of 11 years and 64% were male and 36% female. In 27 families the mother attended, and seven of these also had the father in attendance. In one family it was just the father who attended, without the mother. Some families had other family members like siblings, grandparents, or aunts with them, and in a small number of cases an additional professional.

We video-recorded these naturally occurring real-world mental health assessments so that we could examine what *actually* happens in these environments. We could have interviewed the staff and families retrospectively to ask them about the assessment, but what people think they say and do is often different to what people genuinely say and do. Furthermore, recall relying on memory can be notoriously unreliable. Therefore, the project was designed to look at the actual conversations between practitioners and families and used what is called naturally occurring data (see Kiyimba et al., 2019 for detail). To analyse our data, we used a reflective form of interventionist conversation analysis (see O'Reilly et al., 2020); which is the applied analysis of conversation (talk-in-interaction), because interventionist CA is especially relevant and useful for research in healthcare settings (Barnes, 2019). For those unfamiliar with conversation analysis this is essentially a qualitative method of analysing how people talk to each other, such as the structure and use of words, and ideally suited for looking at naturally occurring data (Sacks, 1992), and specifically we utilised a form of applied conversation analysis (reflective interventionist) because of our partnerships with clinical practitioners, and our commitment to quality improvement (Antaki, 2011; Lester and O'Reilly, 2019; O'Reilly et al., 2020). Transcription of the data therefore used the approach of Jefferson to illustrate *how* things were said as well as what was said (Jefferson, 2004). A guide to this can be found in the introduction to this volume.

As our analysis unfolded and we examined what practitioners are really doing when they perform a mental health assessment there were many things that we noticed. Congruent with the reflective style of the approach, and the partnership style of working with clinical practitioners, we were able to identify many areas of "good practice", where certain communication styles, techniques, or activities really encouraged the children or young people to "open up" and disclose personal detail about their lives or feelings. This micro-approach with its focus on language also enabled us to see aspects of the interaction that did not go so well, where the child refused to answer, got confused, was ignored, or where opportunities to find out more were potentially missed. In the moment, these can be difficult to see, a practitioner engaged in the conversation has to work in real time. However, practitioners in mental health are reflective, open to learning, and generally value opportunities to identify best practices and make changes for quality improvement purposes. Certainly, our open partnership working with clinical practitioners has proved fruitful in understanding the clinical encounter, and in providing useful messages to those working in the field, but also to those who are new to mental health and in clinical training. We provide just a few of our core communication findings in turn, to help identify certain ways that can facilitate the engagement of children or young people and their families in a mental health assessment, and these techniques are certainly translatable to any field where practitioners work with young populations. We start with a common question in assessments: "Why are you here?"

Why are you here?

Understanding why someone attends an appointment sounds obvious but inviting them to tell their story is crucial to patient-centred care. It can be all too easy to turn to a parent and ask them for the reason why they are attending the appointment but appreciating the child or young person's understanding of it can provide useful insights. Through exploring their ideas, concerns, and expectations (Pendleton et al., 1984) the practitioner can appreciate how the individual perceives their situation, enabling them to share their worries and what they hope to gain from the consultation. It is viewed as good practice to explore health beliefs in adults, but it is questionable how often are children's opinions about their health welcomed.

Asking children or young people the question "Why are you here?" should be viewed as a vital step in engagement as it places their views at the centre stage and helps the practitioner understand the problem from their perspective. These types of questions usually appear near the beginning of the session, and function as a way of initiating the institutional business of problem talk (O'Reilly et al., 2015). When a child or young person is asked the reason for attending it treats them as knowledgeable about their condition and allows them greater opportunity to participate in the rest of the session (Tates et al., 2002). In this way, then, the child's knowledge is mobilised in context and makes all subsequent talk "recipient designed" and child focussed. Surprisingly, in our data only about half of the children/ young people were asked for their perspective on why they attended. In some cases, often with younger children the parents were asked first. However, in some instances this also occurred with older children whose parents were engaged instead of them. Consequently, this could lead to the child feeling like a minor part and incidental to what is happening and subsequently disengage from the rest of assessment.

Despite some variation in the phrasing of the question such as "Do you know why you are here?" or "What was your understanding of why you'd come here today?" there were no clear differences in the responses. This is especially interesting as *why*-interrogatives are framed to solicit accounts but may also communicate a stance that the agent is accountable (Bolden and Robinson, 2011). Children and young people's responses fell into three broad categories in terms of accounting for the visit. Some used medical concepts, such as "I think it's OCD"; the so-called "candidate diagnosis" (Stivers, 2002), others used lay terminology such as "something 'bout difficulties". The most common response, however, was to claim in some form that they did now know why they were present themselves. For an overview of these three categories, we refer you to the original article (O'Reilly et al., 2015).

The use of medical or lay terminology may signal how much the child or young person recognises about their "problem". The words used should be treated with caution and it is important to explore meaning from their perspective. Sometimes these replies were shaped by previous encounters for example with health services or what they heard at home or school. These responses allowed a springboard for the practitioner to further explore the child's conceptualisation of their problem through clarification: "Can you tell me a little more about that?" This dialogue facilitates engagement by a shared understanding of the nature of their problem, essentially, they feel listened to. Appreciating the child or young person's understanding of a problem is the basis for agreeing to and engaging with any treatment deemed necessary, and in older children, informed consent. Thus, the practitioner's engagement can demonstrate to the child or young person they are being listened to and illuminate valuing of opinions.

Practitioners need to be aware to taking a response of "I don't know" on face value. In child counselling research, the response "I don't know" was shown to be treated as the child resisting the question rather than not knowing (Hutchby, 2002). Our data illustrated the diverse reasons why the children answered in this way and practitioners' responses were equally different. In some cases, the child later showed that they did not know the reason for attending while in others the child was in fact expressing other feelings such as anxiety or their disdain at having to come to the appointment (e.g., "I just didn't wanna come today"). Practitioners responded either by accepting the child did not know, trying further questions to elicit a response, or alternatively asking the parent instead.

Ironically, "Why are you here?" is often asked in the opening phase of the assessment when the child's anxiety is raised and asking the resistant child why they are there may generate a negative or confrontational reaction. Instead of over-tenacious use of the similar questions, taking a less threatening approach such as the safer question "Okay, so who have you brought with you today?" may put them at ease, helping to engage them. By keeping the dialogue open with the child it may be possible to revisit the reason for attendance in the latter part of the consultation at a point where they feel more engaged with the practitioner. These differences reflect the difficulties of forming a therapeutic relationship. This emphasises the need to firstly work proactively before the session on informing children about the expectations of the session and requires patience, creativity, and perseverance to create an environment which helps engagement and cooperation.

Three wishes

If you really want to engage a child or young person then finding out what matters to them is crucial but may in practice be ignored or discounted. Discovering any patient's agenda can be a complex process and presents certain challenges, but for children and young people an additional element of creativity may be needed. One commonly used technique is a question based on "three wishes", often expressed as "If you had three wishes what would you like to happen?" The institutional function of such a question is to give insight into the child's expectations and ascertaining their goals for the assessment and thus there are certain expectations that the wishes will have relevance to the presenting reasons for attendance. The practitioners thus used this technique as a medium to investigate what was important to the child or young person in respect to their mental health (Kiyimba et al., 2018).

Analysis of the data highlighted several different responses to this question which affected the subsequent interaction. Some responded with answers that were not reflecting the institutional business of the assessment, such as "I want to be rich" or "for JLS [a famous pop group] to live in my house". These types of answers may reflect their age, language ability, or limited insight into their problem. Regardless of the reason, such answers were treated by practitioners as non-relevant to the appointment. It was arguably more successful (in the sense of being goal-oriented), in cases where the child or young person had previously shown an understanding of the reasons for attending the appointment, or if a wish related to the problem, for example "my OCD go away" and "stop being naughty". The practitioner may need to be more explicit in setting the scene before asking the question particularly with those who have learning or neurodevelopmental difficulties where understanding may be more concrete or in cases of the reluctant attendee. The success of this technique hinges on the shared understanding of "Why are you here?" and reflects the engagement of the child or young person in the whole process (we encourage you to read the original paper; Kiyimba et al., 2018).

Subjective units of distress (SUDs)

Rating scales have become ubiquitous as part of modern life; evaluating anything from the quality of service at a restaurant to the attributes of a potential romantic partner. Quantifying emotions in children or young people can be notoriously difficult and rating activities can be used an assessment tool to evaluate of the extent of a child's feelings, such as anger, sadness, or anxiety. One of the most frequently used scales is the Subjective Units of Distress (SUDs) scale as developed by Joseph Wolpe (1969). This is a verbal or visual self-assessment scale which measures the intensity of distress currently or previously experienced by the child or young person, normally on a scale of 0–10. The use of a small range with personalized anchors (e.g., "not at all nervous" for 0 and "very nervous" for 10) is simple and helps ease the decision-making process. Such scales can be further adapted to be age-appropriate and possible visual representations including illustrations on a glass, a thermometer, or a teapot, can be used where the feeling is indicated pictorially.

SUDs are most commonly used for monitoring the therapeutic progress of an intervention but in our context, they acted as an important tool to assess baseline level of functioning at the initial assessment. In this instance, they acted to both qualify as well as quantify the degrees of emotion expressed and experienced. In some instances, they were refined to provide more information about the child's level of distress. SUDs were not only utilised just to assess the current level of feeling but could be fine-tuned to compare the child's experience over a specified time frame or in different settings, such as home and school. Phrases such as "Would that have been different if I had asked you a year ago?" contextualised how recently an emotion had been present in their life. Painting a picture of the fluctuations that occurred in presentation established whether symptoms were improving or worsening "so really you felt a little less happy over the last year". Practitioners often ask questions about the duration of a specific feeling and its relationship to the present and the data highlighted how using SUDs can further refine their responses. For example, greater clarity about how long a certain level of sadness had been experienced by the young person was ascertained by asking "Is that the only time?" and "How long did it stay at three?" The different contexts and situations in which the distress occurs is an important element of the assessment and can be accomplished by asking for ratings of emotions in different environments such as home, school, or even the clinic setting.

We do caution at this point that rating scales may not be entirely accurate in a clinical sense. Our research highlighted the importance of developing a joint understanding between the child and the practitioner as to the meaning of the numbers on the scale. It emerged that valid and more reliable results were more likely when a scale used a single emotion "On a scale of 1–10 with 10 being the most sad, where do you rate yourself now?" rather than a dichotomous scale of contrasting emotions "one is feeling really really sad ten is feeling really really happy". This was important as this allows the nuances of one specific feeling to be expressed in varying degrees (see Kiyimba and O'Reilly 2020).

"You said x" prefaced questions

Asking the right question is at the heart of good communication. "Rubbish in, rubbish out" is an appropriate computer science axiom which implies flawed input produces nonsensical output. In clinical practice this translates to "ask the wrong question, get the wrong answer". Questions do not function just for information gathering but have a wider purpose, for example in clarifying, reflecting, showing interest, and listening. Practitioners tend to use a variety of question styles but there is often a tendency to ask too many. Choosing the right words, in addition to allowing an individual the time to answer are among the skills that foster engagement.

While in our data we examined many different types of question, one specific question type that stood out as facilitating engagement was the "you said x" prefaced question. In Chapter 4, Nikki Kiyimba provides a more in-depth discussion of "you said x" prefaced questions, and here we provide a simple overview as they form part of our key repertoire of findings and communication recommendations. The core concern was that when a child or young person talked about an issue previously in the session, this provided a foundational way for the practitioner to seek further elaboration, especially in more sensitive aspects of the conversation. Specifically, we found that "you said x" prefaced questions were an example of good communication practices in the sense that when these were used, the child or young person disclosed sensitive information and provided more depth than they had previously.

Previous research has shown that children may find it challenging to answer questions about sensitive matters (O'Reilly and Parker 2013). The data showed practitioners used the phrase "you said x" to successfully re-introduce topics previously mentioned by the child or young person. It could also be used to soften a forthcoming question if the phrase "you said x" was followed by either paraphrasing or repeating the exact words the child used. For example, "so when you said that you were going to take a knife to yourself ...", allowed the practitioner to talk about a delicate risk-assessment item of possible suicidal ideation by framing it as something the child had said. If these prefaces are used before a question it was shown to be effective in prompting the child or young person to give further relevant and detailed information about the topic, allowing the practitioner a platform to seek further clarification.

Consider the following example:

Prac: *You used an important word earlier. You said they provoke me.*
Prac: *What happens? How would they provoke you?*
Child: *They start to call me names.*

In this example, the practitioner has reintroduced a topic from earlier in a sensitive manner softening the actual question and encouraged the child to disclose further important information. The value of this technique is that it was shown to be highly effective in our data and is a communication technique that practitioners can easily incorporate into their own work. This sort of strategy is a powerful way of engaging children because it relies on an agreed shared knowledge from the child or young person's domain. The "you said x" technique shows that you have listened to and valued what they are saying. Using their own words is a simple way of bringing their own knowledge back into the conversation and positively affirms the value of their views and perspective. In these kinds of cases, the child or young person always provided more detail about the event and allowed the practitioner to explore it with further questions (see Kiyimba and O'Reilly, 2018). Encouraging children to provide detail about an event or an emotion that is a little more sensitive or might be embarrassing for them to talk about can be a challenge for practitioners. What we demonstrated in our analysis of this phenomenon was that by making a statement of shared knowledge before the specific question promoted open dialogue.

Practical application

In this chapter we have introduced you to some of the central messages and recommendations that have been identified from our close engagement with real-world mental health assessment data. From that, we distil some useful practical tips that you may want to bear in mind when working with children and young people in mental health. We provide these in Box 2.2.

Clinical reflection: Elizabeth McSweeney

Before we move to conclude the chapter, Elizabeth McSweeney reflects on the research:

Health professionals can have differing opinions on the best way to talk to children, something that was highlighted to me on an impromptu hospital visit to our local Children's Accident and Emergency Department with my young daughter. On asking her details by the nurse checking us in, I indicated to my daughter to answer. The nurse looked surprised and took me to one side to question if I really was her mother as I did not appear to know her personal details! Whilst half appreciating her fastidiousness in being alert for safeguarding, I thought seemed a sad reflection on how we value talking to children and that allowing a child to answer a question about themselves was automatically assumed to be a safeguarding issue rather than

---

Box 2.2   Practical tips for communication

Practical tips for improving communication with children in mental health settings

- Talk to the child, it is time well spent – keep the child central to consultation
- Asking the child why they are there is a useful way to assess their understanding of their problem. Do not be afraid to revisit the question later in the assessment if the child is unwilling to engage
- Using the three wishes technique can be a useful way to assess the child's goals and wishes but for maximum effectiveness, make sure they understand the context of the question
- A visual rating scale can be a less threatening way of assessing the level of a child or young person's distress. Remember to assess one emotion per scale
- Using the phrase "you said" can be effective in showing you are listening, reintroduce sensitive topics, or softens a potentially difficult question

the child having some autonomy. Even in a paediatric setting that healthcare professionals may not be used to involving children in their care.

Communication lies at the heart of primary care and in my role as general practitioner the consultation offers me a glimpse into an intimate part of a patient's life. The busy world of every day primary care means juggling many competing demands from formulating a diagnosis and negotiating a shared management plan to establishing rapport and providing patient-centred holistic care often within the confines of a 10-minute appointment. Good communication is key to the success of this and a fundamental part of undergraduate and postgraduate general practice training. Most trainees will be familiar with the concept of how the "golden minute" at the start of the consultation can elicit useful information whilst conveying the sense of being listened to. The importance of establishing "ideas, concerns, and expectations", in other words, discovering the patient's agenda, is something that in ingrained on the brains of all trainees. Many consultation models, such as Pendleton, Neighbour, or Helman have sprung up to internally guide practitioners to incorporate such elements whilst developing their own style of communication and consulting.

Many of our consultations in primary care are with children who attend with anything from a minor infection, acne or more significant developmental or emotional problems. Despite the increased focus on the importance of teaching communication skills in medical education, there is still relatively little focus on teaching communication with children and even less in the art of triadic consulting with clinician, parent, and child. Teaching ways of talking with children is often an afterthought and leaves many clinicians unclear how to communicate effectively with children. The most widely used consultation models in primary care assume a dyadic style of consulting between clinician and adult and there is a dearth of models focused on the needs of children. This may be due to lack of awareness that children have different communication needs or assumptions made the adults, clinician, or parent, that there is not any real need to talk to the children, or that even young children have views and wish to be heard. Often after the cursory question or two to the child the entire consultation may often be with the parent where the child can appear to be a passive passenger to the whole experience and the limits of a short consultation time only serves to perpetuate this.

Although this research is derived from a specialist mental health setting, the findings are applicable across a wide range of settings and different situations where children are present and addresses some of the difficulties in consulting with children, and gaps in training, identified in primary care. This research makes clear that children want to, and should be, active participants in their own healthcare. If we are to be truly child-centred, we should be engaging with the parent but also with the child. We cannot use techniques predicated on adult ways of interacting and need to actively adapt our consulting styles to the needs of the child. This is particularly true for children presenting with emotional or mental health problems where feeling heard and being allowed to participate may be crucial to their overall engagement in discussing topics that may be painful or engaging with treatments that may be difficult.

This research highlights simple yet effective ways to adapt how we consult to more effectively engage and involve children. Asking the child rather than the accompanying adult why they are here can help with establishing the child's understanding of the situation, their own opinions or wishes, or highlight reluctance they might have in attending. Asking the child for three wishes, while at the same time knowing how to ask and how to interpret the responses, is eminently suitable for the shorter consultation and further discovering the agenda. Using "you said" as a way of coming back to potentially difficult subjects may seem obvious but appears to work. On many occasions, children have found it difficult to quantify their feelings and the idea of using an analogue scale to get the most reliable answers also seems efficient.

Overall considering the specific issues around communicating with children these techniques and others can create a more child-friendly environment and the increasing need to respect their role in decision making. Short consultation times remain one of the challenges in primary care and one of many constraints when talking to children. However, while these techniques may require a change in consulting style, they are simple, do not take additional time, and are easy to incorporate into our everyday busy consultations with children and into teaching programmes for undergraduate and postgraduate medical training.

Discussion

Despite the trend in healthcare towards "state-of-the-art" equipment and technology, extensive investigations, or complex treatments, the power of words remains an underrated therapeutic tool for working with children, young people, and families. Effective mental health assessments, diagnosis, and treatments are very dependent on the credibility and trust built and the outcomes of clinical practice are better when children and young people are appropriately engaged in the whole process. It is increasingly recognised in health, education, and social care settings that children and young people should be involved in their care, but in practical terms this can often be difficult to achieve. However, recognising that they are experts in themselves makes them feel a key part of the process and understanding the problem from the perspective of the child or young person allows the practitioner insight into their worries or fear, their expectations, and their experiences and this facilitates building realistic and meaningful goals. Surprisingly, although there has been some research into communication, the literature around children (especially those with mental health conditions), remains sparse. Video recording first assessments was innovative and creative, and opened a window into what really transpires in a child mental health assessment. The advantages of this type of research is that the analysis is based upon the authenticity of a real-life encounter rather than relying on retrospective accounts.

In this chapter, the data represented relatively small snippets of the interactions but when weaved together into an assessment they helped to reveal the tapestry of the child or young person's story. The observations we have presented here highlighted how the use of words can help to ensure the child or young person is central to process, may encourage detailed responses to sensitive questions or could demonstrate listening and valuing of their opinion and not just simply a means for the practitioner to collate information. The concepts cited in this chapter may sound deceptively simple in approach, but they had a powerful effect on influencing the trajectory of the assessment and subsequent level of engagement and involvement of the child or young person. They are rooted in everyday language and understandable to all parties. Although the data originated from a specialist secondary care setting, the messages about communication are relevant and applicable to a much broader audience and can be utilised by anyone working with younger populations.

Observing and analysing real-life interactions enable the findings to become relevant to training for those new to clinical practice, or experienced practitioners developing further skills. The assumption is that communication is an intrinsic "soft skill" for most practitioners, which is often given lower priority in training programmes and while it may be taught to some extent, for most professionals, personal development depends on ad-hoc experience. The acquisition of skills in communication would benefit from a firmer evidence base to provide a more consistent foundation to develop clinical practice. The lack of prioritising of communication research reinforces the misguided conception that communication is not important. Furthermore, it is assumed that more experienced practitioners do not need continued training in this area with the belief that they already have those skills and yet, in reality, they get very little feedback. Although most clinical practitioners are reflective, it is evident from our observations that everyone can benefit from further development of their communication skills. Reflection and, ideally, being observed should encourage a higher proficiency in all areas of communication, but having evidence is arguably more persuasive to those who may be resistant to changing their practice.

To conclude, we remind you that recognising that children are not mini-adults is important given the changes to our understanding of the spectrum of childhood and in an age of child-centred practice and children's rights it is necessary to engage children in their own care. Engagement of children and young people is a multi-faceted process and in the real world it can become peripheral to the needs of any of the adults in the room. The careful use of words and the powerful influence of the meanings of those words we choose can have an expressive and long-standing impact on how we work with younger populations and the outcomes we all seek.

References

Antaki, C., 2011. Six kinds of applied conversation analysis. In: Antaki, C. (Ed.), *Applied Conversation Analysis: Intervention and Change in Institutional Talk.* Palgrave MacMillan, Hampshire, pp. 1–4.

Balint, M., 1957. *The Doctor, His Patient and the Illness.* Churchill Livingstone.

Barnes, R., 2019. Conversation analysis of communication in medical care: description and beyond. *Res. Lang. Soc. Interact. 52* (3), 300–315.

Bor, W., Dean, A., Najman, J., Hayatbakhsh, R., 2014. Are child and adolescent mental health problems increasing in the 21st century? A systematic review. *Australian N. Zeal J. Psychiatry 48* (7), 606–616.

Bolden, G., Robinson, J., 2011. Soliciting accounts with *why*-interrogatives in conversation. *J. Commun. 61*, 94–119.

Buston, K., 2002. Adolescents with mental health problems: What do they say about health services? *J. Adolescence 25*, 231–242.

Cahill, P., Papageorgiou, A., 2007. Triadic communication in the primary care paediatric consultation: A review of the literature. *Br. J. Gen. Pract. 57*, 904–911.

Centor, R., 2007. To be a great physician, you must understand the whole story. *Medscape Gen. Med. 9* (1), 59.

Chu, B., Kendall, P., 2004. Positive associations of child involvement and treatment outcome within a manual-based cognitive behavioral treatment with anxiety. *J. Consulting Clin. Psychol. 72*, 821–829.

Dallos, R., Draper, R., 2010. *An Introduction to Family Therapy: Systemic Theory and Practice* (third ed.). Open University Press, Berkshire.

Day, C., Michelson, D., Hassan, I., 2011. Child and adolescent service experience (CHaSE): Measuring service quality and therapeutic process. *Br. J. Clin. Psychol. 50*, 452–464.

Dogra, N., Parkin, A., Gale, F., Frake, C. (2017) *A Multidisciplinary Handbook of Child and Adolescent Mental Health for Front-Line Professionals* (third ed.). Jessica Kingsley Publishers, London.

Hutchby, I., 2002. Resisting the incitement to talk in child counselling: aspects of the utterance 'I don't know'. *Discourse Stud. 4* (2), 147–168.

Hutchby, I., 2010. 'Active listening': formulations and the elicitation of feelings-talk in child counselling. *Res. Lang. Soc. Interact. 38* (3), 303–329.

Jefferson, G., 2004. Glossary of transcript symbols with an introduction. In: Lerner, G.H. (Ed.), *Conversation Analysis: Studies from the First Generation.* John Benjamins, Amsterdam, pp. 13–31.

Kiyimba, N., Lester, J., O'Reilly, M., 2019. *Using Naturally Occurring Data in Health Research: A Practical Guide.* Springer, Germany.

Kiyimba, N., O'Reilly, M., 2018. Reflecting on what 'you said' as a way of re-introducing difficult topics in child mental health assessments. *Child. Adolesc. Ment. Health 23* (3), 148–154.

Kiyimba, N., O'Reilly, M., Lester, J., 2018. Agenda setting with children using the three wishes technique. *J. Child. Health Care 22* (3), 419–432.

Kiyimba, N., O'Reilly, M., 2020. The clinical use of Subjective Units of Distress scales (SUDs) in child mental health assessments: A thematic evaluation. *J. Ment. Health 29* (4), 418–423.

Lester, J., O'Reilly, M., 2019. *Applied Conversation Analysis: Social Interaction in Institutional Settings.* SAGE, Thousand Oaks, CA.

Lewis, C., Rachelefsky, G., Lewis, M., de la Sota, A., Kaplan, M., 1984. Randomized trial of A.C.T. (Asthma Care Training) for kids. *Pediatrics 74*, 478–486.

Mash, E.J., Hunsley, J., 2005. Special section: developing guidelines for the evidence-based assessment of child and adolescent disorders. *J. Child. Adolesc. Psychol. 34* (3), 362–379.

NHS Digital, 2018. Mental health of children and young people in England, 2017: Summary of key findings. https://files.digital.nhs.uk/F6/A5706C/MHCYP %202017%20Summary.pdf (accessed 11.12.18).

O'Reilly, M., Karim, K., Stafford, V., Hutchby, I., 2015. Identifying the interactional processes in the first assessments in child mental health. *Child. Adolesc. Ment. Health 20* (4), 195–201.

O'Reilly, M., Kiyimba, N., Lester, J., Muskett, T., 2020. Reflective interventionist conversation analysis. *Discourse & Communication 14* (6), 19–34.

O'Reilly, M., Parker, N., 2013. 'You can take a horse to water, but you can't make it drink': exploring children's engagement and resistance in family therapy. *Contemporary Family Ther. 35* (3), 491–507.

Pendleton, D., Schofield, T., Tate, P., Havelock, P., 1984. *The Consultation: An Approach to Learning and Teaching.* Oxford University Press, Oxford.

Persson, S., Hagquist, C., Michelson, D., 2017. Young voices in mental health and care: exploring children's and adolescents' service experiences and preferences. *Clin. Child. Psychol. Psychiatry 22* (1), 140–151.

Sacks, H., 1992. *Lectures on Conversation (Vols. I & II, edited by G. Jefferson).* Basil Blackwell, Oxford.

Stafford, V., Hutchby, I., Karim, K., O'Reilly, M., 2016. 'Why are you here?' Seeking children's accounts of their presentation to CAMHS. *Clinical Child Psychology and Psychiatry 21* (1), 3–18.

Stivers, T., 2002. Presenting the problem in pediatric encounters: 'symptoms only' versus 'candidate diagnosis' presentations. *Health Commun. 14* (3), 299–338.

Strong, T., Busch, R., Couture, S., 2008. Conversational evidence in therapeutic dialogue. *J. Marital. Family Ther. 34* (3), 388–405.

Tates, K., Meeuwesen, L., Bensing, J., Elber, E., 2002. Joking or decision making? affective and instrumental behaviour in doctor–patient parent communication. *Psychol. Health 17*, 281–295.

Tseliou, E., Burck, C., Forbat, E., Strong, T., O'Reilly, M., 2020. The discursive performance of change pocess in systemic and constructionist therapies: A systematic meta-synthesis review of in-session therapy discourse. *Family Process.* doi:10.1111/famp.12560.

United Nations Convention on the Rights of the Child, 1989. Conventions on the Rights of the Child. London: UNICEF. http://www.unicef.org.uk/Documents/ Publicationpdfs/UNCRC_PRESS200910web.pdf (accessed 07.12.19).

Wolpe, J., 1969. *The Practice of Behavior Therapy.* Pergamon Press, New York.

Chapter 3

Exploring the practical potential of discursive research in family therapy

Olga Smoliak, Shari Couture, Joaquin Gaete Silva, Marnie Rogers-de Jong, Ines Sametband, and Andrea LaMarre

Introduction

Talking is central to psychotherapy; psychotherapy itself has been described as a "talking cure" dating back to Freud (Marx, Benecke, and Gumz, 2017). While researchers and therapists have pointed out that talking is not the only aspect of therapy that contributes to therapeutic processes and outcomes (e.g., Benecke, Peham, and Bänninger-Huber, 2005; Tschacher, Rees, and Ramseyer, 2014), talking remains the primary way of "doing" therapy (Marx et al., 2017). In family therapy, especially, talking can provide the route through which families' concerns, experiences, and relationships are articulated, made sense of, and transformed. While there are frameworks delineating how talk therapy works (e.g., Marx et al., 2017), there is room to explore the communicative and interactional aspects of how therapeutic change comes about – that is, how change is produced *through* talking and interacting.

Discursive approaches (e.g., discourse analysis, conversation analysis, critical discourse analysis) can help clarify the taken for granted means through which clients and therapists use language to accomplish therapeutic goals. Beyond a focus on the content of language, which is shared across most approaches to therapy, discursive approaches direct one's attention to the process of therapists and clients talking together, that is, to how language is put to use and what gets accomplished through such use. The focus is on how questions are asked and responded to and how therapists join clients to manage professional agendas (e.g., for clients to shift away from mutual blaming to seeing their problems as rooted in their relational dynamics). Many therapists see language as either irrelevant to their work or as a medium of communication peripheral to the "real work" of therapy, which is presumed to transpire within clients or in their relational dynamics. Discursive approaches advance a different view of therapeutic change as transpiring through language use. Therapy talk is seen as *producing* alternative psychological or relational realities, not merely communicating or *reflecting* therapeutic processes occurring outside and beyond language use.

In this chapter, we will use the terms "discursive approaches," "discursive inquiry," and "discursive analysis" interchangeably. In our use of each term, we intend to offer a discussion of the merit of their common focus: the process conversational participants negotiate as they accomplish the work of therapy. Discursive inquiry entered family therapy in the 1980s (e.g., Gale, 1991; Gale and Newfield, 1992) and has experienced steady growth, evidenced by a proliferation of book chapters, methodological reviews, published studies, and special issues devoted to discursive work (e.g., O'Reilly et al., 2018; Tseliou, 2013; Tseliou and Borsca, 2018). Our overall aim in this chapter is to propose that discursive inquiry offers relevant and valuable knowledge to practitioners. Specifically, we discuss and illustrate how discursive inquiry can be useful to family therapists in addressing common practical dilemmas they may encounter in their work with families. We offer a brief description of discursive research methods and a selective review of how they can be applied to study family therapy.

Context and literature review

Discursive approaches

Discursive approaches share the premise that clients' psychological and relational "reality" is not given, singular, or stable but created through social practices and interactions. Within the broad umbrella of discursive approaches to research, there are varied and multiple orientations to "discourse"; each strand has distinct aims, premises, and procedures. Conversation analysis (CA) is used to investigate how social interaction is organized in turn-by-turn linguistic sequences (e.g., Schegloff, 2007; Sidnell and Stivers, 2013). It lends itself to "micro" analysis of language that could, for example, highlight how asking a question in a certain way opens up or closes down what can be said in response. Maynard's (1991) work offers a specific example of this. He used CA to illustrate how medical practitioners tend to deliver a medical diagnosis in an indirect way. This research showed how practitioners elicited clients' perspectives on their concerns and then fit their diagnoses within clients' descriptions and explanations. Maynard argued that this way of sequencing the delivery of a diagnosis helps bridge the gap between the doctor's and the client's views and increase the likelihood that the diagnosis is accepted by the client.

Discourse analysis (DA) and discursive psychology (DP) tend to focus on how language is used in real-life situations. DP scholars investigate how people practically manage and use psychological concepts (e.g., emotion, memory, agency, intent) and to what social, interactional aims (e.g., blaming, convincing, refusing) (e.g., Edwards and Potter, 1992; Potter, 2012). An example of a DP study is Edwards' (1999) analysis of couple counselling. For

Edwards, emotion words are not the mirror image of inner emotional states but are rhetorical devices used by speakers. The same emotion word can be mobilized to accomplish different social actions in interaction. Edwards showed how one partner, Connie, described her partner Jimmy's emotions of anger and jealousy as inherent aspects of Jimmy's identity (i.e., he is a jealous and aggressive person). Jimmy, in contrast, described his anger not as a personality predisposition but as a sensible response to Connie's recurrent provocations – her ongoing flirting with other men. The study highlights that DP offers a discursive antidote to conventional psychological conceptions of emotions as invariable internal states.

In contrast to micro-oriented approaches that amplify what happens at the level of concrete speaking turns, critical discourse analysis (CDA) takes a broader view, examining links between power and language. CDA's focus is on how societal power relations are established, reproduced, and/or resisted in and through talk and text (e.g., Wodak and Meyer, 2015). Sutherland et al.'s (2016) analysis of couple therapy offers an example of a CDA study. The researchers showed how partners in intimate relationships described their partner roles and obligations with reference to broader (normative or dominant) cultural prescriptions concerning gender and sexuality (e.g., there are only two genders, men should do X and women should do Y, men's sexual desire is privileged). They also highlighted how therapists can reinforce (and challenge) normative gender and sexuality through their responses to partners' descriptions.

Each of these approaches offers insight into the nuances of language and its use in therapy. In order to argue and illustrate the relevance and value of discursive research for practitioners, we focus here on three practical questions or dilemmas family therapists commonly face when working with families. These are:

1. How to help families move beyond "conversational impasses" where family members seem to be stuck speaking from different or incommensurable ways of understanding their situation.
2. How to challenge or augment views presented as singular or ultimately correct (without being heard as blaming or critical).
3. How to advance professional knowledge collaboratively or in ways that do not negate or disregard clients' familiar understandings and preferences.

We offer conversational strategies that may help therapists to address these questions and dilemmas. We present extracts from various discursive studies, which in our view, help demonstrate the value of attending to discourse in formulating solutions to the aforementioned dilemmas. To select extracts, we reviewed existing discursive studies of psychotherapy to identify moments of interaction that can, in our view, capture the dilemmas we list above. Most examples we present come from initial sessions of family therapy, which are often concerned with "problem for-mulation," or therapy participants co-developing and negotiating de-scriptions and understandings of concerns that bring families to therapy (e.g., what is "wrong" and who is responsible). Issues of blame and ac-countability, therefore, seem central in these initial therapeutic encounters and feature throughout our discussion.

For the purposes of illuminating specific discursive "strategies" or prac-tices that will help therapists in their work, we focus on micro-oriented approaches to discourse analysis, namely CA and DA. However, it is im-portant to note that CDA studies can provide key insights for therapists, particularly into the lives of clients living in a world that constructs them as problematic (think, for instance, of racist, sexist, ableist, and other "isms" that limit people's possibilities for flourishing). Thus, while it is beyond the scope of our chapter to speak in depth to CDA studies, we draw the reader's attention to studies of therapy that unpack sexist (e.g., Sutherland et al., 2016; Sutherland et al., 2017), neoliberalist (e.g., LaMarre et al., 2019), and biomedical discourses (e.g., Gaete et al., 2017; Sutherland et al., 2016).

Research conclusions

Addressing conversational impasses

Family therapists often encounter different or even opposite accounts of family difficulties. Commonly, different members in a family position one family member (e.g., a child or one partner) as the source of problems or as someone to blame. Family members may expect therapists to join and validate their specific versions of "what is wrong" and "who is at fault." However, the therapist's role is to be "neutral," or not to take sides (or better, to take *all* sides; Anderson, 1997). Thus, family therapists have the delicate task of balancing all views within the family, while inviting families to move beyond blame and individually focused explanations.

At times, family members can get stuck in a conversational "impasse" when each member is overly invested in their way of understanding a topic. Family therapists are often aware of how a particular view may contribute to the "impasse" by inviting defensiveness in another family member or other unintended relational consequences. Finding a com-promise, or a mutually agreed-upon way of understanding and addres-sing an issue, may not be easy. Arguably, it is difficult to move forward beyond an impasse unless all views are "put on the table" and treated as valid and legitimate. Several strategies can be identified in the discursive literature for moving beyond these impasses. We will delineate selected strategies below. They include using questions, obliqueness, orchestrated talk, and humour.

Open-ended and closed-ended questions

How might family therapists begin to move past these seemingly in-surmountable forks in the therapeutic road? It is here that discursive ap-proaches can help to illustrate ways forward. Couture's conversation analytic work on conversational impasses (e.g., Couture, 2006, 2007; Couture and Sutherland, 2006) clarifies how it may be possible to establish all views as valid and to facilitate a shared way forward on a specific issue in a conversation.

In practice, this may look like engaging family members with different perspectives together in renegotiating their views in an attempt to find a middle ground (Couture, 2006). In her work, Couture (2006) shows an in-teraction between Joe, an adolescent struggling with depression and sui-cidality, and his parents. Joe had just left the hospital where he had signed a therapeutic contract that stated he would keep himself safe. At the beginning of the session (not shown), the parents spoke from a position of certainty that Joe would follow through with the contract, while Joe conveyed doubt in his ability to uphold the contract. This position of certainty may con-stitute a kind of pressure and be counterproductive, potentially setting Joe up for failure. From a systemic-relational perspective, it is the "coupling" of extreme doubt and certainty that may keep families stuck in conflictual interactions and impasse. Both positions may need to be explored and challenged.

Exemplar 1 (from Couture, 2006, p. 291), (J- Joe, B - Bob, T- therapist)

```
01. T:    >Okay< (.7) um (1.2) now how do you feel about this like is
02.       this is something you feel that you can live or (.5) or are
          you not
03.       sure that you can live up to this or not er:: (3.4)
04. J:    >I don't know< (.4) I don't know yet I guess (.)
05. B:    ((Bob furrows brow))
06. T:    Don't know ya (1.2) well that is probably an honest
          statement
07.       because you don't know for sure right? (.)
08. J:    *Mhmm* (.)
```

Here, the therapist demonstrates neutral engagement by eliciting Joe's per-spective on the contract instead of joining the parents' view that Joe can (and should) follow the contract. The therapist asks an *open-ended question* ("how do you feel about this," line 1), seeking Joe's perspective on the matter at hand (the safety contract). Interestingly, before Joe has an op-portunity to answer the question, the therapist reformulates the question into a more closed-ended (Yes or No) question (lines 2–3). The new question changes what Joe can say in response. Whereas the open-ended question *(how do you ...)* seeks information from Joe, the closed-ended questions merely asks Joe to confirm or disconfirm what the therapist says. That is, with the latter the therapist (not Joe) becomes the source of an alternative, disagreeing idea. The design of the reformulated question is noteworthy ("is this is something you feel that you can live or (.5) or are you not sure that you can live up to this or not"). The question delineates two possible views on the contract: Joe adhering to its conditions (the parents' position) and Joe struggling to commit or "live up" to the contract (an alternative position). It may be a way to put on the table all family members' views and not take a stance (i.e., remain a neutral party). Joe may feel pressured to adopt the parents' version. The yes/no question asks Joe to merely confirm the therapist's guess rather than be the one to introduce a different view. It may be a way to bring forth all family members' views, especially views that may be marginalized within families.

In the extract, we can see the discursive workings of managing accountability. For instance, Joe manages accountability as he responds to this invitation, selecting an uncertain position with regard to his capacity to follow through ("I don't know < (.4) I don't know yet I guess (.)"). This response may reflect the stakes for Joe. If he commits to the contract, he may be kept accountable if he fails to live up to it (e.g., his parents may later say "you promised"). On the other hand, if he says he will not live up to the contract, he may get opposition or criticism from his parents. In using the adverb "yet" in response to these questions, Joe manages to overcome the dilemma by not committing to the contract but not explicitly opposing his parents. The therapist acknowledges ("Don't know ya") and accounts for Joe's claimed lack of knowledge ("well that is probably an honest statement because you don't know for sure right?", lines 6–7). In so doing, the therapist treats Joe's perspective as legitimate. Couture's work illustrates the possibilities of discursive research for identifying ways that therapists can use language to surface varied points of view and remain neutral.

Obliqueness, orchestrated talk, and humour

As differing positions are elicited and developed as valid within the conversation, where do therapists go from there? Conversational analytic work by Aronsson and Cederborg (1996) illustrates conversational practices used by therapists to navigate the therapist's neutral engagement or the development of "equidistance between opposing parties in family therapy talk" (p. 208). Aronsson and Cederborg analysed a session in which a therapist helped bring forth two opposing perspectives within the family: that a teenage son (Sam) is ready to move out and live on his own (Sam's father's position) and that he is not yet mature and responsible enough to move out (Sam's mother's position). Sam's position is ambiguous: there are benefits and disadvantages to living on his own. The therapist used a series of discursive strategies, including "orchestrated talk" (inviting family members to directly speak to each other), humour, and "obliqueness" (i.e., impersonal constructions such as "one" or "people"). These strategies were used to advance specific views in therapy without appearing to blame certain family members. Exemplar 2 demonstrates the use of humour and orchestrated talk. The dynamic of protectiveness and overprotectiveness within the family is explored. The mother is worried about and protective of Sam. At the same time, the relational dynamic is explored of Sam feeling the obligation to stay home to take care of his parents and their distress and conflict.

Exemplar 2 (M - mother, T - therapist).

```
01. M:   (talks about her husband) He does pick on me, yes, he does
         pick on
02.      me, but mostly it's about Sam that he picks on me
03. T:   You see, I do think there's an issue here, in the same way
         that I
04.      think Sam needs to be able to tell you that he can manage
         on his
05.      own, I think you may need to tell Sam that you can manage
         on your
06.      own.
07. M:   Oh right, yes.
08. T:   If you think you can. Otherwise you need to keep him en-
         gaged as your
09.      protector for the next 10 years.
10. M:   (to Sam) I don't think that's necessary darling, I do
         think we
11.      can manage.
12. S:   It is a very awkward position for me like.
13. T:   Wait a minute, were you convinced by what she said?
14. S:   No.
```

The therapist organizes or *orchestrates talk* between the family members, inviting them to say specific things to each other ("I think you may need to tell Sam that you ..."). The issue of Sam struggling to become more independent is framed not as Sam's issue but as rooted in relational dynamics and involving actions of both parties (the parents and Sam). The suggestion may be received by the mother as implying that she is to blame. The humorous packaging of the suggestion (lines 5–6) can be used to mitigate criticism of the mother and address "the issue of protection and overprotection without getting involved as anyone's ally" (Aronsson and Cederborg, 1996, p. 207). The example above shows how multiple, conflicting views can be brought forth while downplaying the therapist's alignment with specific family members.

In this section, we have explored how discursive methods can draw our attention to how different points of view are established as valid, and how therapists can invite family members to transcend conversational impasses. Impasses occur when family members struggle to negotiate between different views. However, the conflictual issues families bring to therapy are not limited to impasses. Families may experience relational challenges when there is stagnation of meaning, that is, specific views get established as the only "correct" way to understand a matter at hand (e.g., how to parent, relate to each other, spend family time, accomplish specific tasks). Meanings that are established as singular within families may or may not be a part of a relational or interactional impasse, depending on how others respond (e.g., endorse, resist, concede) to views promoted as ultimately correct or singular. In the next section, we engage with discursive work on practices that therapists can use to challenge and augment singular explanations and foster multiplicity and diversity of viewpoints.

Challenging singular views

Indirect challenges, neutral language, and contextualization

Early work in DA from Burck et al. (1998) illustrates communicative practices used by therapists to challenge views presented as singular or superior. Burck et al. conducted a case study involving parents, Brenda and Miles, who presented in family therapy with concerns related to parenting their three children. The parents described themselves as "parenting negatively" (all quoted speech in this section comes from Burck et al., 1998). It can be a delicate matter for therapists to offer alternative views, as they may be heard as implying that clients' ideas are inadequate or insufficient. One way to augment and diversify perspectives in therapy conversations is to *indirectly challenge* clients' views by eliciting alternative meanings from other family members. In response to Brenda's self-blame in describing herself as a parent (e.g., "I am a failure," "... a lot of the time I am very cross"), the therapist elicits Miles' perspective on their parenting. Miles undermines the idea that they are fully responsible and deserve blame, which challenges Brenda's initial description of herself as a "bad" parent. By introducing alternative, even contradictory, points of view into the room, space is opened up for multiple versions of "reality" to co-exist.

Therapists can also use language to acknowledge a client's version without accepting its negative evaluation. Burck et al. (1998) described how the father, Miles, presented himself as "failing" as a parent due to experiencing "low-grade depression" that interferes with his ability to set boundaries with the children ("... I take the easy option"). The therapist challenges Miles' negative evaluation of himself as a parent ("… easy option") using morally *neutral language*, implying that his parenting approach is different rather than inferior or problematic ("well, it's a *different* one isn't it"). In so doing, the therapist acknowledges Miles' version while not aligning with his negative evaluation of his parenting. The therapist then goes on treating Miles' self-deprecatory/blaming account as problematic by offering a relational framing of the "problem." He describes Miles' "(over) easy" approach not as a result of his depression, but of his efforts to compensate for Brenda being "(over)hard" as a parent.

Burck et al. (1998) provide another example of the therapist refusing to join the clients' individually focused self-deprecating appraisals. The therapist had inferred that Brenda had a history of abuse as a child. When she tells a story that paints herself as crazy or "paranoid," the therapist *contextualizes* Brenda's actions and replaces Brenda's negative self-evaluation with an alternative that frames her response as "quite reasonable" (the therapist's words) given the context of her life. By replacing "bad" with "reasonable," the therapist was able to challenge a dominant self-deprecatory view. In all, this pioneering study of Burck et al. (1998) illustrates three discursive strategies to reframe unhelpful (e.g., blaming, self-deprecatory) dominant views, namely: by indirect challenges (inviting competing views from others), using neutral language, and contextualizing.

Advancing professional knowledge in "resistance-informed" ways

Clients' disagreements

As professionals, therapists are often seen as experts on clients' psychological or relational concerns and how to remedy them. A shift toward postmodern, collaborative family therapy practice (e.g., Anderson, 1997; McNamee and Gergen, 1992; White and Epston, 1990) raises questions about how therapists can use their professional authority to facilitate change in ways that attend to and give space for clients' knowledge and agency. Postmodern therapists challenge the notion of an expert therapist and strive to collaborate and *co*-construct meanings with clients, rather than seek clients' compliance with professionals' meanings.

From a discursive (CA) perspective, power and collaboration are understood as constituted and negotiated between parties in therapeutic interactions, rather than as unilateral moves (Boden and Zimmerman, 1991; Roy-Chowdhury, 2003). While therapists may promote ideas, families can "resist" or push back against therapists' descriptions and meanings. By "resisting" we mean clients disagreeing, questioning, or displaying other (more subtle) ways of not taking up therapists' offerings. We favour therapy practice that is informed by resistance from clients. Therapists can modify their offerings and work together with clients to co-develop more mutually endorsed descriptions. For example, clients may resist being portrayed as an inferior parent (O'Reilly and Lester, 2016); as responsible for their family's presenting problems (Patrika and Tseliou, 2016); as competent and resourceful (MacMartin, 2008); or as not abiding by local cultural norms (Sametband and Strong, 2018). Clients sometimes show clear disagreement, such as by replying "No" or "I disagree." But because disagreeing can be a sensitive matter (Pomerantz, 1984), particularly given authority or "expertise" culturally attributed to therapists, clients often push back in subtler ways. Collaborative therapists try to work in ways that are "resistance-informed" (de Shazer, 1984). For example, they may pause when observing clients hesitate in their response to them and become curious about the act of hesitating itself. They may recognize these moments and treat them as opportunities for renegotiating meanings. In this way, we have reframed resistance, moving from the more traditional pathologizing of client actions towards valuing and respecting these important client offerings.

Exemplar 3 (taken from MacMartin, 2008) illustrates how clients' resistance (e.g., disagreement, reluctance to accept ideas, or interest in joining a proposed description or direction) to therapists' ideas can manifest in interaction. The client talks about an incident when she was able to assert herself with her ex-partner in the relationship in which she has felt controlled and disempowered.

Exemplar 3 (T – therapist, C – client)

```
01. T:   How does it feel tuh (0.3) sort of see a-where you
         have been
02.      (0.5) °exerting yer influence. an an having control
         over (him).°
03.      (0.7)
04. C:   Feels good but then I wonder. °why can't I apply it to::°
05.      (0.6) other areas (0.3) with him.
```

We see an example of a so-called "presuppositional question" (MacMartin, 2008) on lines 1–2. Presuppositional questions advance specific ideas. Rather than presenting their ideas as declarative statements, speakers may embed them within questions. By directly answering presuppositional questions, their recipients implicitly endorse or take up the questioner's ideas. In Exemplar 3, the therapist asks the question that embeds "optimistic" presuppositions about clients (e.g., their capacities, competencies, qualities). Optimistic questions are used in solution-focused therapy to highlight clients' resourcefulness and competencies (MacMartin, 2008). The question advances the notion of the client as someone who has more agency and power in her relationship and presents the client's action as an example of a pattern (*have been…*). The client affiliates ("Feels good") with the therapist's view of her having greater power and agency in her relationship but then produces a disagreeing response ("but then I wonder..."). She downgrades the optimism embedded in the therapist's question by limiting the scope of her influence over her ex-partner ("°why can't I apply it to:: (0.6) other areas (0.3) with him.°", lines 4–5). In so doing, the client displays that the therapist's view of her does not fully "fit." With the more traditional notion of resistance, the client's response could be considered a "roadblock" to therapeutic progress. From our resistance-informed discursive lens, aware-ness of this subtle disagreement can be an opportunity for the therapist to further develop the description of the client that would be mutually deemed "adequate." Again, often clients disagree in subtle ways without producing an overt disagreement. Therapists may benefit from sensitizing themselves to various manifestations of clients' resistance and how they respond. In this way, discursive research is a useful resource for enhancing therapists' awareness and reflexivity.

Implications for therapy research

It has been argued that therapy needs to be guided by the available scientific evidence of effective practice (Yates, 2013). Evidence-based practice in psychotherapy has become equated with an attempt to develop a list of empirically supported therapies for specific mental disorders (Chambless and Ollendick, 2000). Some have argued that this dichotomous under-standing of effective therapies (either supported or unsupported) is overly restrictive and simplistic, and that evidence-based practice is greater than a list of empirically supported therapies (Westen and Bradley, 2005). Narrow conceptualizations of evidence not only exclude potentially efficacious therapeutic approaches that do not easily lend themselves to more con-ventional methods of inquiry but may also contribute to a gap between science and practice by privileging artificial and highly controlled over real-life practice settings (Berg, 2019).

By examining therapy naturalistically as it unfolds in real-world settings, discursive research offers practice-based evidence, or evidence that is close to "actual" practice (Barkham and Mellor-Clark, 2000). It provides a distinct, conversational kind of evidence of helpful (and less helpful) ways of working with clients (Strong et al., 2008; Helps, this volume). Because discursive research examines in-session conversational evidence it can help clarify how therapists can practice in responsive ways, or ways informed by emerging responses from clients. Discursive methods of inquiry are not meant to re-place more conventional ways of studying therapy but to complement them (Tseliou, 2018). Arguably, no single method can answer all possible ques-tions about therapy.

Discursive methods are especially well-suited for the study of family therapy concerned with *relationships* among family members and between family members and therapists (Tseliou, 2018). Discursive scholars attend to both the broader context of meaning-making in family therapy and the immediate interactional context. Each therapy participant's contribution to an interaction is seen as shaped by and shaping the actions and responses of their co-participants (Heritage, 1984). Within family therapy, discursive methods align particularly well with the concerns and premises of social constructionist therapies (e.g., narrative, solution-focused, collaborative), which are focused on meaning co-construction in therapy and on how power dynamics in a society shape and constrain clients' self-definitions, experiences, and relationships. Thus, practicing family therapists can learn from this kind of evidence, and we make some suggestions for practice in Box 3.1.

Box 3.1   Practical tips

Practical tips for improving communication

- Reading or conducting discursive studies can help practitioners identify discursive practices involved in the actual "doing" of therapy (e.g., asking and responding to specific kinds of questions). Therapists can attempt to apply this discursive knowledge in their own work with clients and observe the immediate interactional effects of their communicative efforts.
- When thinking about "discourse" and its analysis, remember that discourse can involve micro-level attention to language (e.g., turns of phrase, the way questions are asked, turn-taking, etc.) and broader-level constructions (e.g., discourses or commonly relied upon ways of describing people or things)
- Some questions for therapists to consider:
  - How do family members respond to each other?
  - What may be signs that their responses to each other are limiting rather than facilitating their conversation?
  - What assumptions about family members and relational dynamics seem to be at play in the interaction and how are they interactionally produced and advanced?
  - How do family members respond to my initiatives in our conversation?
  - How can I notice times when what I offer does not seem to "fit" for clients, and collaboratively generate and renegotiate descriptions so they are more mutually agreeable?
  - What do family members' responses tell me about a conversation's direction? Is this direction coherent with the client's expressed or displayed agendas and preferences?

Reflections: Implications for therapy practice

"In order to find the real artichoke, we divested it of its leaves." (Wittgenstein, 1953, aphorism 164)

Learning about and conducting discursive research has shaped our work as therapists in significant ways. Wittgenstein's aphorism inspires us in adopting a critical stance towards more conventional approaches to the study of therapy, which too often treat communication as an "add-on" to the real work of therapy – very much like how we may illusorily aim to find the real artichoke by taking away all its leaves. Most therapy researchers envision therapeutic phenomena (e.g., change, distress, relationships, self) as existing beyond and outside of language. Therapists' and clients' language (e.g., post-therapy reports, in-session interactions) are implicitly treated as a window into the heart of therapy. In contrast, as discursive scholars, once we came to see therapy *as* communication, it seemed relevant to focus on it analytically. Discursive therapy research treats language not as a resource to "get at" processes and outcomes of therapy but as a topic in its own right (Zimmerman and Pollner, 1970). Conventional systemic and psychological notions seemed much less mysterious when approached as *conversational accomplishments* of therapists and clients (Sutherland et al., 2013). For us, notions like therapeutic "impasses" can be seen as conversational stucknesses such as the patterns of blaming-defending that we showcased in this chapter. And therapists may unwittingly be recruited into participating within them – or critically and artfully resist such invitations by engaging in alternative, more "therapeutic" conversational practices. Through a discursive lens, such practices become observable and learnable.

From this view, we have transformed the question of "What's *the* problem in this family?" into the following inquiries: "How are particular understandings or versions of the problem produced, what are the potential implications on clients (and broader professional practice and society) of advancing these versions, and which alternative understandings are we disregarding?" Discursive inquiry helped us become better sensitized to important aspects of our interactions with clients (Madill, 2015; Tseliou, 2018) and develop discursive awareness and resourcefulness (Strong, 2016). Through reading and conducting discursive studies, we were able to "step back from communications in order to see what is constructed in and from them" (Strong, 2016, p. 481).

Early in our development as therapists, we noticed that our textbooks and courses often emphasized what therapists were supposed to say or do. It seemed as though if we talked in some particular way (e.g., "That must have been tough"), clients would inevitably understand that we were performing certain actions, such as showing empathy or validating their experiences. We soon realized that therapy interactions do not necessarily go as expected; our conversations with families were dynamic and sometimes unpredictable.

Conducting discursive research provided us with a useful framework to look closely at the details of our interactions, including how clients responded to our intended interventions with minute verbal and non-verbal cues. We learned to slow down and check in with clients when their responses informed us that we may have missed something important. Discursive research methods have also helped us look closely at the dominant cultural ideas informing clients' (and our) lives, attend to broader structures of oppression, and invite families to move beyond gender, racial, and other stereotypes (McDowell et al., 2018; McGoldrick and Hardy, 2019). We feel better equipped to recognize times when we may be using our position as family therapists to "impose" our own ideas rather than collaborate with clients to create and negotiate understandings that are mutually agreeable. As such, adopting this framework has enabled us to take a more critical, reflexive stance on our practice, with greater awareness of how power can be enacted and challenged in therapy conversations (Guilfoyle, 2003).

From the family therapy literature, we learned that it is important for us to remain neutral and not side with selected family members. We were less clear about how to implement a neutral stance. Discursive inquiry offered possible conversational means of maintaining a neutral stance. We learned, for example, that speaking in generalities (e.g., "Some people find that ... Often this is what happens ...") may be a way to challenge certain views or introduce alternative views without leaving clients feeling blamed or criticized. We also learned that rather than responding to clients ourselves (e.g., challenging, disagreeing, offering alternatives), we could ask others in the family to respond to them and build on their responses or introduce alternative views.

Conclusion

In this chapter, we have highlighted key strategies identified in the discursive literature that can help therapists to identify how linguistic practices can, quite literally, change therapeutic practice. By taking a reflexive stance on language use in therapy, therapists can effectively navigate challenges like remaining neutral in the face of conflicting points of view and challenging culturally dominant or singular perspectives. Discursive approaches are often explicitly power-conscious and contextual; they allow for thoughtful engagement with how what happens in the therapy room interacts with context and cultures in the broader world. We have made several suggestions throughout the chapter for further reading, should readers become interested in broadening their lens on therapeutic practice to integrate awareness of discourse. We hope this chapter presents exciting grounds on which to build deeper understandings of how what we say has material impacts on therapeutic encounters and the broader systems in which they are situated.

References

Anderson, H., 1997. *Conversation, Language, and Possibilities: A Postmodern Approach to Therapy.* Basic Books, New York.

Aronsson, K., Cederborg, A., 1996. Coming of age in family therapy talk: Perspective setting in multiparty problem formulations. *Discourse Process 21* (2), 191–212. doi:10.1080/01638539609544955.

Barkham, M., Mellor-Clark, J., 2000. Rigour and relevance: Practice-based evidence in the psychological therapies. In: Rowland, N., Goss, S. (Eds.), *Evidence-Based Counselling and Psychological Therapies.* Routledge, London, pp. 127–144.

Benecke, C., Peham, D., Bänninger-Huber, E., 2005. Nonverbal relationship regulation in psychotherapy. *Psychotherapy Res. 15*, 81–90. doi:10.1080/10503300512331327065.

Berg, E., 2019. How does evidence-based practice in psychology work? – As an ethical demarcation. *Philos. Psychol. 32* (6), 853–873.

Boden, D., Zimmerman, D., 1991. *Talk and Social Studies in Ethnomethodology and Conversation Analysis.* Polity Press, Cambridge.

Burck, C., Frosh, S., Strickland-Clark, L., Morgan, K., 1998. The process of enabling change: A study of therapist interventions in family therapy. *J. Family Ther. 20*, 253–267. doi:10.1111/1467-6427.00086.

Chambless, D., Ollendick, T., 2000. Empirically supported psychological interventions: Controversies and evidence. *Annu. Rev. Psychol. 52*, 685–716. doi:10.1146/annurev.psych.52.1.685.

Couture, S., 2006. Transcending a differend: Studying therapeutic processes conversationally. *Contemporary Family Ther. 28*, 285–302. doi:10.1007/s10591-006-9011-1.

Couture, S., 2007. Multiparty talk in family therapy: Complexity breeds opportunity. *J. Systemic Therapies 26* (1), 63–82. doi:10.1521/jsyt.2007.26.1.63.

Couture, S., Sutherland, O., 2006. Giving advice on advice-giving: A conversation analysis of Karl Tomm's practice. *J. Marital. Family Ther. 32* (3), 329–344. doi:10.1111/j.1752-0606.2006.tb01610.x.

de Shazer, S., 1984. The death of resistance. *Family Process 23*, 11–21. doi:10.1111/j.1545-5300.1984.00011.x.

Diorinou, M., Tseliou, E., 2014. Studying circular questioning "in situ": Discourse analysis of a first systemic family therapy session. *J. Marital. Family Ther. 40* (1), 106–121. doi:10.1111/jmft.12005.

Edwards, D., 1999. Emotion discourse. *Cult. Psychol. 5* (3), 271–291. doi:10.1177/1354067X9953001.

Edwards, D., Potter, J., 1992. *Discursive Psychology.* SAGE, London.

Gaete, J., Sametband, I., St. George, S., Wulff, D., Tomm, K., Durán, G., 2018, Early view: Realizing relational preferences through transforming interpersonal patterns. *Family Process.* doi: 10.1111/famp.12417.

Gaete, J., Smoliak, O., Couture, S., Strong, T., 2017. DSM diagnosis and social justice: Inviting counselor reflexivity: discourse in practice. In: Audet, C., Pare, D. (Eds.), *Social Justice and Counseling.* Taylor & Francis, Routledge, New York, pp. 197–212.

Gale, J., 1991. *Conversation Analysis of Therapeutic Discourse.* Ablex, Norwood, NJ.

Gale, J., Newfield, N., 1992. A conversation analysis of a solution-focused marital therapy session. *J. Marital. Family Ther. 18* (2), 153–165. doi:10.1111/j.1752-0606.1992.tb00926.x.

Guilfoyle, M., 2003. Dialogue and power: A critical analysis of power in dialogical therapy. *Family Process 42*, 331–343. doi:10.1111/j.1545-5300.2003.00331.x.

Heritage, J., 1984. *Garfinkel and Ethnomethodology*. Polity, Cambridge.

Kogan, S., Gale, J., 2007. Decentering therapy: Textual analysis of a narrative therapy session. *Family Process 36* (2), 101–126. doi:10.1111/j.1545-5300.1997.00101.x.

LaMarre, A., Smoliak, O., Cool, C., Kinavey, H., Hardt, L., 2019. The normal, improving and productive self: Unpacking neoliberal governmentality in therapeutic interactions. *J. Constructivist Psychol. 32* (3), 236–253. doi:10.1080/10720537.2018.1477080.

MacMartin, C., 2008. Resisting optimistic questions in narrative and solution-focused therapies. In: Perakyla, A., Antaki, C., Vehvilainen, S., Leudar, I. (Eds.), *Conversation Analysis and Psychotherapy*. Cambridge University Press, New York, pp. 80–99.

Madill, A., 2015. Conversation analysis and psychotherapy process research. In: Gelo, C.G., Pritz, A., Rieken, B. (Eds.), *Psychotherapy Research: Foundations, Process, and Outcome*. Springer, New York, pp. 501–515.

Marx, C., Benecke, C., Gumz, A., 2017. Talking cure models: A framework of analysis. *Concept. Anal. 8*, Art. 1589. doi:10.3389/fpsyg.2017.01589.

Maynard, D., 1991. The perspective-display series and the delivery and receipt of diagnostic news. In: Boden, D., Zimmerman, D.H. (Eds.), *Talk and Social Structure: Studies in Ethnomethodology and Conversation Analysis*. Polity, Cambridge, pp. 164–194.

McDowell, T., Knudson-Martin, C., Bermudez, J., 2018. *Socioculturally Attuned Family Therapy*. Routledge, New York.

McGoldrick, M., Hardy, K., 2019. *Re-visioning Family Therapy: Addressing Diversity in Clinical Practice* (third ed.). Guilford, New York.

McNamee, S., Gergen, K.J. (Eds.), 1992. *Therapy as Social Construction*. SAGE, London.

Muntigl, P., Choi, K., 2010. Not remembering as a practical epistemic resource in couples therapy. *Discourse Stud. 12*, 331–356. doi:10.1177/1461445609358516.

Muntigl, P., Horvath, A., 2016. A conversation analytic study of building and repairing the alliance in family therapy. *J. Family Ther. 38*, 102–119. doi:10.1111/1467-6427.12109.

O'Reilly, M., 2015. "We're here to get you sorted": Parental perceptions of the purpose, progression and outcomes of family therapy. *J. Family Ther. 37*, 322–342. doi:10.1111/1467-6427.12004.

O'Reilly, M., Kiyimba, N., Lester, J., 2018. Discursive psychology as a method of analysis for the study of couple and family therapy. *J. Marital. Family Ther. 44* (3), 409–425. doi:10.1111/jmft.12288.

O'Reilly, M., Lester, J., 2016. Building a case for good parenting in a family therapy systemic environment: Resisting blame and accounting for children's behaviour. *J. Family Therapy 38* (4), 491–511. doi:10.1111/1467-6427.12094.

O'Reilly, M., Parker, N., 2013. "You can take a horse to water but you can't make it drink": Exploring children's engagement and resistance in family therapy. *Contemporary Family Ther. 35*, 491–507. doi:10.1007/s10591-012-9220-8.

Patrika, P., Tseliou, E., 2016. Blame, responsibility and systemic neutrality: A discourse analysis methodology to the study of family therapy problem talk. *J. Family Ther. 38* (4), 467–490. doi:10.1111/1467-6427.12076.

Pomerantz, A., 1984. Agreeing and disagreeing with assessments: Some features of preferred/dispreferred turn shapes. In: Atkinson, M., Heritage, J. (Eds.), *Structures of Social Action.* Cambridge University Press, Cambridge, pp. 47–101.

Potter, J., 2012. Discursive psychology and discourse analysis. In: Gee, J.P., Handford, M., *The Routledge Handbook of Discourse Analysis.* Routledge, pp. 104–119.

Roy-Chowdhury, S., 2003. Knowing the unknowable: what constitutes evidence in family therapy? *J. Family Ther. 25* (1), 64–85. doi:10.1111/1467-6427.00235.

Sametband, I., Strong, T., 2018. Immigrant family members negotiating preferred cultural identities in family therapy conversations: A discursive analysis. *J. Family Ther. 40* (2), 201–223. doi:10.1111/1467-6427.12164.

Schegloff, E., 2007. *Sequence Organization in Interaction: A Primer in Conversation Analysis.* Cambridge University Press, Cambridge.

Sidnell, J., Stivers, T., 2013. *The Handbook of Conversation Analysis.* Blackwell, New York.

Stancombe, J., White, S., 1997. Notes on the tenacity of therapeutic presuppositions in process research: Examining the artfulness of blamings in family therapy. *J. Family Ther. 19*, 21–41. doi:10.1111/1467-6427.00036.

Strong, T., 2016. Discursive awareness and resourcefulness: Bringing discursive researchers into closer dialogue with discursive therapists? In: O'Reilly, M., Lester, J. (Eds.), *The Palgrave Handbook of Adult Mental Health: Discourse and Conversation Studies.* Palgrave Macmillan, London, pp. 481–501.

Strong, T., Busch, R., Couture, S., 2008. Conversational evidence in therapeutic dialogue. *J. Marital. Family Ther. 34* (3), 388–405. doi:10.1111/j.1752-0606.2008. 00079.x.

Strong, T., Tomm, K., 2007. Family therapy as re-coordinating and moving on together. *J. Systemic Therapies 26* (2), 42–54.

Sutherland, O., LaMarre, A., Rice, C., Hardt, L., Jeffery, N., 2016. Gendered patterns of interaction: A Foucauldian discourse analysis of couple therapy. *Contemporary Family Ther. 38*, 385–399. doi:10.1007/s10591-016-9394-6.

Sutherland, O., LaMarre, A., Rice, C., Hardt, L., Le Couteur, A., 2017. New sexism in couple therapy: A discourse analysis. *Family Process 56* (3), 686–700. doi:10. 1111/famp.12292.

Sutherland, O., Sametband, I., Silva, J., Couture, S., Strong, T., 2013. Conversational perspective of therapeutic outcomes: The importance of preference in the development of discourse. *Counsel. Psychother. Res. 13* (3), 220–226. doi:10. 1080/14733145.2012.742917.

Sutherland, O., Strong, T., 2011. Therapeutic collaboration: A conversation analysis of constructionist therapy. *J. Family Ther. 33*, 256–278. doi:10.1111/j.1467-6427. 2010.00500.x.

Tschacher, W., Rees, G., Ramseyer, F., 2014. Nonverbal synchrony and affect in dyadic interactions. *Front. Psychol. 5*, 1323. doi:10.3389/fpsyg.2014.01323.

Tseliou, E., 2013. A critical methodological review of discourse and conversation analysis studies of family therapy. *Family Process. 52* (4), 653–672. doi:10.1111/ famp.12043.

Tseliou, E., 2018. Conversation analysis, discourse analysis and psychotherapy research: Overview and methodological potential. In: Smoliak, O., Strong, T. (Eds), *Therapy as Discourse: Practice and Research*. Palgrave Macmillan, New York, pp. 163–186.

Tseliou, E., Borsca, M., 2018. Discursive methodologies for couple and family therapy research: Editorial to special section. *J. Marital. Family Ther. 44* (3), 375–385. doi:10.1111/jmft.12308.

Weatherall, A., Gibson, M., 2015. "I'm going to ask you a very strange question": A conversation analytic case study of the miracle technique in solution-based therapy. *Qualitative Res. Psychol. 12* (2), 162–181. doi:10.1080/14780887.2014.948979.

Westen, D., Bradley, R., 2005. Empirically supported complexity: Rethinking evidence-based practice in psychotherapy. *Curr. Directions Psychological Sci. 14* (5), 266–271. doi:10.1111/j.0963-7214.2005.00378.x.

White, M., Epston, D., 1990. *Narrative Means to Therapeutic Ends*. W. W. Norton, New York.

Wittgenstein, L., 1953. *Philosophical Investigations* (G.E.M. Anscombe, Trans.). Blackwell, New York.

Wodak, R., Meyer, M., 2015. *Methods of Critical Discourse Studies* (third ed.). SAGE, London.

Yates, C., 2013. Evidence-based practice: The components, history, and process. *Counselling Outcome Res. Evaluation 4* (1), 41–54. doi:10.1177/2150137812472193.

Zimmerman, D.H., Pollner, M., 1970. The everyday world as a phenomenon. In: Douglas, J. (Ed.), *Understanding Everyday Life*. Aldine, Chicago, pp. 80–104.

Chapter 4

Communication in clinical psychology
Using "you said" in interactions with children to assess for risk

Nikki Kiyimba

Introduction

For those working with children and young people the scenario of asking a question and being met with a shoulder shrug or "I don't know" or "nothing" as a response will be familiar. This chapter will focus on one aspect of communicating with a child or young person, which is the use of "you said" at the start of a sentence, which can act as a precursor to asking a question. This has been found to be particularly effective as a starting point, so that the follow-up question is usually effective in eliciting an appropriate and relevant answer. The research study described in this chapter is the first of its kind to examine how healthcare practitioners use this approach when working with children. Using "you said" in conversation is a bit like when people report what *another* person has said using "he said" or "she said" at the start of the sentence. When people repeat what another person has said in this way, it is called "reported speech". Reported speech is recognisable by: a) the speaker tries to say it in the same as the way it was said by the person being referred to, through intonation and volume or accent etc. and b) what is reported is usually prefaced with the phrase "he said" or "she said" (Holt, 1996). An example might be that the staff team is gathered to discuss what a client has said when that client is not present. One staff member might choose to "report" it; "she said 'I have two sisters who live nearby' ". The words of the client are spoken as if they are an exact replication of what the client said.

In reported speech the person whose words are being replicated is usually not present (but may be). The words that are being quoted as they were spoken by someone other than those who are present, and in a different place at an earlier time. However, when people use the phrase "you said" they do so in the present moment, when they are talking *to* the person whose words they are repeating. Because of this difference, a distinction in terminology is used, and the phrase "reflected speech" has been created to refer to interactions using "you said", as distinct from "reported speech" interactions that generally start with "he said" or "she said" (Kiyimba and

O'Reilly, 2018). Although this chapter is authored from the perspective of a clinical psychologist, reflected speech is not a specific technique that is a unique part of that training. In fact, its use is found across various professional and ordinary interactions. It may be something that you have noticed already that people do when they are talking to each other. What this chapter aims to do is to show its use in a systematic way through a piece of research based on data collected from a series of child and adolescent mental health assessments. Looking at its properties in a systematic way using transcripts of actual live assessments helps to show more clearly how sentences with "you said" are constructed, and how effective they can be. This is particularly relevant in situations where "difficult" topics such as those related to shame, trauma, or risk are important to explore. Before discussing the findings of the research project that this investigation is based on in more detail (Kiyimba and O'Reilly, 2018), a brief overview of the research setting and current literature on asking children questions is provided.

Research setting and literature

The setting for this piece of research was the collection of data from 28 families attending a child and adolescent mental health (CAMHS) clinic in the UK. In these meetings their child was being assessed by a team of mental health professionals to decide whether the child required specialist psychological therapy or other specialist support for their reported mental health difficulties. The allocated time for these assessments is typically about 90 minutes, and a great deal of information needs to be gathered during that time for the mental health team to make an accurate assessment of the child's needs and appropriate service provision. Although the primary purpose of assessments is to screen for mental health difficulties in children (Parkin et al., 2003), another function is relationship building with the family and child or young person. It is therefore important for the assessing team to ask the right kinds of questions that will provide them with the right kind of information to make that decision, whilst at the same time developing and maintaining a positive relationship. Consequently, the requirements of the task of information-gathering need to be considered within the context of this being the first time that the team has met the family and child or young person. Additionally, children often report feeling quite anxious prior to attending CAMHS appointments (Bone et al., 2014), and so how to address sensitive topics may be challenging.

Typically, the assessing team will ask questions to the parents/guardians or other family members and will also try to gather information from the child or young person themselves (see Karim et al., this volume). Previous research has shown that it is important to engage directly with children in this process, and not just rely on parents' reports, as this involvement of children leads to better outcomes (Chu and Kendall, 2004). Depending on the age and the presenting difficulties of the child or young person being assessed, the need for skilful questioning is crucial to the success of this endeavour. This may in part be due to the resistance that some children can exhibit in institutional encounters, which can be challenging to manage (Hutchby, 2002). In part it may also be because children can find it difficult to respond to "personal" questions when in unfamiliar environments (Parker and O'Reilly, 2013). Furthermore, where there are particularly delicate or sensitive topics that need to be addressed relating to the institutional business, these discussions can be potentially troublesome and delicate to navigate (Antaki, 2007). The complexity of a child mental health assessment where there are family members present ought not to be underestimated, as this can significantly affect the capacity of all participants to articulate their responses to the questions asked. In turn these dynamics necessarily have an impact on the kinds of utterances that are made available to the clinician to potentially draw upon later as part of a "you said" formulation. As a result, professionals can find it quite difficult to find ways to ask questions of children that are effective in providing them with useful information (Stivers, 2001).

Due to the nature of institutional settings, there is frequently a necessity to collect quite a bit of information, and questions are naturally the most time-efficient way of focusing on gathering the information required (O'Reilly et al., 2015). However, given the unfamiliarity of the environment, the anxiety that family members may have about being assessed, and the potentially sensitive of difficult topics that may need to be addressed, it is important to find ways to gather the required information without it feeling like an interrogation. Thus, the ability to notice and to avoid "rupture" or dis-alignment between professionals and their clients is an important skill to develop (Voutilainen, Peräkylä, and Ruusuvuori, 2010; Parker and O'Reilly, 2013). This means finding ways to ask questions that are effective in gathering the required information, whilst at the same time building and maintaining a good relational level of rapport that will put the clients sufficiently at ease that they feel able to answer the questions asked. Interestingly, one function that the "you said" sequence can accomplish in these environments is to mitigate the power differentials existing between the clinician and family and the clinician and child. However, although question use and design is so important to this process, there is little research to date that has focused specifically on how to ask questions in psychotherapy (Ziolkowska, 2009; MacMartin, 2008: Weatherall and Gibson, 2015; see also, on the difference between question-driven and formulation-driven psychotherapies Peräkylä, 2013).

The research on question use that has been conducted so far has tended to use a type of qualitative methodology called discourse analysis (DA). This is an umbrella term that includes several specific types of research methodology that focus on language use, and often use naturally occurring data to explore institutional discourse practices. Naturally occurring data are pre-existing verbal and textual activities used for research purposes, in contrast to "researcher generated" data such as interviews and focus groups (Kiyimba, et al., 2019). One advantage of using naturally occurring data rather than researcher generated data is that it has more field validity because it has been collected in the context of real-world interaction.

Thus, naturally occurring data are excellent for examining institutional processes and for identifying examples of actual practice rather than relying on subjective retrospective reports. In the case of child and adolescent mental health assessments, having recordings of the actual conversation in real time is invaluable for assessing and evaluating how particular questions are formulated, and their effectiveness in information gathering. This is better than trying to collect retrospective reports through interviews or focus groups (Potter, 2002). Research using a DA approach to analysing naturally occurring mental health CAMHS assessments has already shown that mental health professionals use a number of different ways to ask questions (O'Reilly et al., 2015; Kiyimba and O'Reilly, 2018; Weatherall and Gibson, 2015). This research methodology has also shown that often assessments require that questions are asked in sequences or as a series of questions, as the professionals involved seek to incrementally clarify mental health need (McCabe et al., 2002; Antaki and O'Reilly, 2014). It is therefore timely that understandings of possible ways in which to craft questions to both maintain alignment and engagement with children and young people, and simultaneously acquire relevant information is anticipated to be of interest to a range of professionals.

The investigation reported on here was designed to look a little closer at which kinds of questions were more effective, and particularly how questions that were prefaced by "you said" statements worked in practice. Our research team found that "you said" functioned both to reintroduce a previous topic and provide a platform for asking follow-up questions based on that topic. Through analysis of the data we also discovered consistent features to how reflected speech was introduced (Kiyimba and O'Reilly, 2018). In the present chapter, I will consider the implications of these findings for clinical practice.

Analysis and findings

The 28 video-recorded naturally occurring child mental health assessments that were collected for this research project were analysed using a type of discourse analysis called conversation analysis (CA), and specifically utilised a reflective form of applied CA (see O'Reilly et al., 2020). This is a rigorous and well-established way to investigate the details of how people talk to one another (Heritage, 1984). Although the original data were video recordings, these were transcribed into a written format using a detailed system which includes verbatim words as well as using different symbols to represent emphasis, intonation, volume and timed pauses (Jefferson, 2004). The analysis of the transcripts in CA was inductive (bottom up) and involved first collecting instances of similar types of practices that re-occurred throughout the data set. In this approach, findings from the data are then recorded from the directly observable characteristics of the way that people talk, rather than subjective interpretations (Drew, Chatwin, and Collins, 2001). To enhance the objectivity and rigour of this process, these characteristics were evaluated together by several researchers in the team to ensure credibility and accuracy.

Core findings

By using conversation analysis to investigate the data, it was found that there was a recurrent three-part sequence. The first two parts were:

1. A sentence including the phrase "you said" plus the reflected speech (the professional speaking).
2. A space where the recipient may or may not respond to part one (the opportunity for the client to respond).
   The initial "you said" plus the reflected speech part was observed to propose what was the current shared knowledge between the professional and the client. Depending on whether there was a form of agreement about that proposed knowledge from the client in this space, the third part of the sequence may then be produced, which was:
3. A follow-up question from the professional and answer from the client.

The importance of this third part of the sequence is that the production of the final question and answer was only made possible by the fact that the first two parts were present as a foundation (Kiyimba and O'Reilly, 2018).

Data examples

The following data extract is an example of this three-part sequence. An explanation of how each part maps onto what the Clinical Psychologist and the Child say to one another is provided in Box 4.1, following the extract:

Extract one: Family ten (CP = Clinical Psychologist)[1]

```
1. CP:     you used an im↓portant word earlier you said er they
2.            provoke ↓me
3.            (0.78)
4. CP:     um w w- what ↓happens how would they pro↓voke you?
5. Child:  they: start to ↓call me names
```

Box 4.1   Explanation of how the three part 'you said' sequence maps onto data extract one

Part one: The 'you said' preface plus reflected speech part is seen in lines 1 and 2 when the clinical psychologist says "you said er they provoke ↓me"

Part two: In line 3 there is an opportunity for the child to agree or disagree with the proposed reflected speech that the child had said that they were being 'provoked'. In this space there is a pause of 0.78 seconds. Where there is no resistance or denial, the statement is *treated as* accepted by the child as a true basis for continuing. Notably this is only apparent by looking at the third part.

Part three: The clinical psychologist offers a follow-up question based on what is treated as an agreement from the child that they were being provoked. The question asks for further clarification on that topic in line 4 by asking "what happens, how would they provoke you?" This question then successfully elicits an answer from the child in line 5: "They start to call me names".

Following part one of the sequence, "you said er they provoke me" there was a significant pause "(0.78)". In CA, where there are naturally occurring opportunities within the conversation for another person to speak, these are known as transition relevance places (TRP) (Sacks et al., 1978). One of the ways that these are recognisable is by the "completing" intonation used by the person speaking just before the TRP. In the sequence that I have presented, downward intonation (marked by a downward arrow – ↓me) is one way of representing completing intonation. At this point I have referred to this recognisable opportunity for the child to respond as a recipient response slot. In some instances, the child responded, and at other times (such as this instance) they did not. In this data set where the recipient remained silent at a TRP within a "you said" sequence, this was treated by the speaker as tacit agreement, evidenced by the "next turn proof procedure". The next turn proof procedure is defined as "observing how speakers display in their sequentially 'next' turns an understanding of what the 'prior' turn was about" (Hutchby and Wooffitt, 1999, p. 15). In this data typically, the speaker in the third part of the sequence treated the child's silence in the previous turn as agreement, evidenced by their continuation with further questioning along the same thematic lines.

Taking a clinical rather than conversation analytic perspective on this process, the clinician's speculation about what is being thought and experienced by the child in terms of agreement, is what informs the clinician's transition from stage two to stage three of the sequence. This may rely to some extent on clinical judgment that the child has given assent to the proposition reflected back to the child as indeed being a basis for continuation with a line of questioning on that re-introduced topic. Now that we have seen in the data how silence in part two of the sequence operates, the following extract provides an example of a child verbally agreeing to the proposition made through the "you said" reflected speech in part one of the sequence. Again, a brief explanation is provided in Box 4.2 after the data extract to demonstrate which parts of the data example match with which parts of the "you said" question and answer sequence that is being presented.

Extract two: Family one (CPN = Community Psychiatric Nurse)

```
1. CPN:      I'm ju↑st wo:↑ndering thou↓gh coz you (.) you
2.           said in the: (.) interview room that (.) it
3.           sta↑rted a couple of years ago [it FIRST]=
4. Child:                               [yeah its]
5. CPN:      = ever >st[arted] a couple of years ago<=
6. Child:              [yeah]
```

Box 4.2   Explanation of how the three part 'you said' sequence maps onto data extract two

Part one: The 'you said' preface plus reflected speech part is seen in lines 1 to 3 when the CPN said "you said in the: (.) interview room that (.) It sta↑rted a couple of years ago"

Part two: In lines 4 and 6 there is an opportunity for the child to agree or disagree with the proposed reflected speech about the problem starting a couple of years ago. In both spaces the child agrees by saying "yeah" in overlap with what the CPN is still saying. When people agree in overlap like this it can be a sign of "supportive interaction" (White, 2003, p.13) or strong agreement.

Part three: The CPN asks a follow-up question in line 7 based on the child's agreement about the reflected speech part: "so why↑ do you think it started the↓n?". Quite a full answer is then provided by the child in lines 8 to 11 when they explain what their thoughts are on why the problems started at that particular time, because it was due to: "changing thi:ngs", "chan↑ ging schools".

```
 7. CPN:      = so why↑ do you think it it started the↓n?
 8. Child:    January it could be sorting out changing
 9.           thi:ngs(0.70) I th↓ink it could be like (.)
10.           say↑ing me (.) is coz like (.) I dunno (0.63)
11.           chan↑ging schools an th↓at li↓ke
```

Extracts one and two have been provided to explain exactly how the sequence works, as the rest of the discussion in this chapter hinges on an understanding of how these three parts link together and are mutually dependent upon one another. As this foundation has now been laid, the following extract will not be dismantled in the same way but is provided instead to show how important this conversational device might be in assessing risk. Obviously assessing and managing risk is one of the most important roles that many professionals undertake, and therefore if we can find ways to ask questions about risk in ways that are most supportive and facilitative of eliciting critical information, the value of that is self-evident.

Extract three: Family six (Psy = Psychiatrist)

```
1.   Psy:      so when you ↓said that you were going to take
2.             a ↓knife to yourself
3.             (0.99)
4.   Psy:      yeah?
5.             (1.15)
6.   Psy:      what were you ↓hoping would happen?
7.   Child:    erm (2.45) f::or me to ↓actually kill my↓self
```

The psychiatrist in this assessment used "you said" to reflect to the child a comment made previously about using a knife on themselves (lines 1 and 2). As with extracts one and two, the second part of the sequence is an opportunity for the child to agree or disagree with this proposal (line 3). Furthermore, an agreement is clearly sought by the psychiatrist in line 4 when they add the tag question "yeah" to their proposal. It is inferred therefore that the pause and lack of verbal response from the child after this agreement is sought is treated as tacit agreement. This is evidenced using the next turn proof procedure by the fact that the psychiatrist continues in line 6 with the follow-up question that asks for what the child's intention was in this act of self-harm "what were you ↓hoping would happen?". This follow-up question becomes possible to be asked at this point because the topic of self-harm is now clearly "on the table" as a matter for further discussion. The scene setting and preparation that the "you said" reflected speech part of the extract facilitates, appears to be crucial to providing a shared space where further elaboration about the child's motives for this act can legitimately be sought. In fact the success of this whole sequence is demonstrated in the child's response which clearly outlines their intentionality in line 7, "f::or me to ↓actually kill my↓self". This extract is a powerful reminder of how important it is to formulate questions in ways in which children and young people feel able to answer, so that matters of risk can be appropriately detected and dealt with.

The functional value of using reflected speech in question design

The research on reflected speech presented in this chapter was found to serve several functions. These are listed below and discussed in turn in more detail:

1. to make relevant the re-introduction of a specific topic
2. to provide a platform for a follow-up question in a way that is less challenging
3. to elicit elaboration and/or clarification (Kiyimba and O'Reilly, 2018).

Re-introduction of a topic

Although several topics may have been covered prior to a section of conversation where reflected speech is used, the first function of its use is to select from the previous part of the conversation a specific part of a topic to re-introduce and make relevant again. This means that the speaker (in this case the professional) has some control over the choice of what is put back on the table for further discussion, whilst at the same time not appearing to have been unilaterally decided by the professional. Reflected speech can take the form of a paraphrase or the reproduction of the exact words that were used by a client (Kiyimba and O'Reilly, 2018), in this case the proposition is made using the client's own words. The upshot is that instead of a power display of who gets to choose what things are discussed, using the "you said" reflected speech formulation, the choice of topic is presented as a joint concern.

To provide a platform for a follow-up question

It is possible that if a professional chose to ask a question outright about a particular topic of concern or interest without the preliminary foundation of reporting reflected speech, that the question might feel like a challenge to the client, especially if it related to a sensitive, risk-related, or personal issue. What is shown from the use of the "you said" plus the reflected speech precursor, is that this acts as an agreed foundation or agreed premise from which further questions may be asked. By agreeing (or assenting non-verbally) to the proposed reflected speech, the client in effect allows this re-introduced topic to form the basis for further discussion. It appears that the reflected speech part is experienced by the client as a preliminary type question that projects the likelihood of some further inquiry being forthcoming. It is suggested that it is this initial "agreement in principle" function of reflected speech supports or provides a platform for the follow-up question to be more effective than it might otherwise have been.

To elicit elaboration and/or clarification

The third function of the "you said" reflected speech sequence that was observed in the research was that it ultimately served to prompt an opportunity to ask a follow-up question. The follow-up question enabled the clinician to seek elaboration or more detail or further clarification about what had previously been mentioned by the client about that topic. In other words, by reintroducing an earlier topic, the sequence facilitated an opportunity to talk more about that issue. The fact that all 108 instances of this sequence that were identified in the data resulted in a "successful" outcome in terms of the child or young person providing an appropriate answer demonstrates its effectiveness.

Evidence-based practice

In settings where it is important to gather accurate information, effective questioning strategies are vital to fulfil this objective. What is meant by "effective" in this context is that the client offers a response to the professional's question in the third part of the sequence that is both appropriate and relevant and provides enough detail. In this research project, in each instance "you said" prefaced sequences were effective in gaining further information. Relative to the practical implications of these findings, the research that this study was based on was within the context of a mental health assessment with children and young people, and therefore its primary application would first of all be relevant to that setting. However, it is likely that this type of questioning device is relevant and applicable across several other settings and professional contexts with adults as well and children (Parker, 2003). Based on this, then, I offer some practical tips in Box 4.3.

From a purely pragmatic point of view in terms of the resource constraints that many services are subject to, it is important that staff have skills

---

Box 4.3   Practical tips

Practical tips for improving communication

- Think about the impact of how questions are asked and how effective they are in eliciting appropriate responses
- Consider how using reflected speech in your professional context may support you in this process

to use strategies that are most effective in gathering necessary information. It is hoped that the lessons learned from this piece of research can help professionals to be more considered, and thus more effective in their question design. By using the client's own words in reflected speech, whatever the task at hand, it is also possible for professionals to work in a more client-centred way that demonstrates their attentiveness to the client's narrative. When the reflected speech of the client's own words is reintroduced as a topic, this provides a platform for the professional to ask further questions or seek clarification or elaboration without seeming presumptuous, or that the question is coming from *their* agenda per se. In effect, by using the client's own words, the topic is presented as the *client's* concern, and is treated therefore as a permissible line of enquiry. This can contribute to mitigating the power differentials that exist between the clinician and family and the clinician and child. Therefore, the modulation of this element may be a key factor underpinning the clinical choice to use reflected speech, especially when engaging in the important task of risk assessments.

Practice reflections

It has been an interest of mine for some time to consider the use of "you said" as a conversational device for re-introducing topics, since I first became aware of it in my PhD research into family therapy interactions (Parker, 2003). It was very interesting for me to see again the same patterns occurring in the CAMHS assessment data that this chapter reports on that I had seen in the family therapy data. Also, in my current role as counsellor educator I am often required to assess videos of trainees in practice, and to review the transcripts of their counselling sessions (see Helps, this volume for further discussion of this practice). In these sessions I am intrigued to often notice their use of "you said" during their counselling interactions. From my knowledge of counselling training and clinical psychology training, this is not a specific technique that is taught, and yet I see it being used in practice. As both a discourse analyst and a healthcare professional I value the opportunity to be able to look at how the research I am involved in can be applied to a real world setting, and vice versa to see real world examples of the things that have become research interests. In the literature, these two things are referred to as evidence-based practice and practice-based evidence respectively. The two inform one another – research informs practice, and practice stimulates and informs research.

What I find particularly interesting about "you said" as a tool in conversations that involve sensitive issues such as addictions or risk or shame or trauma, is that it feels more collaborative in practice to introduce the topic as something that the client themselves has already identified they wish to discuss, rather than being a topic that is being unilaterally imposed onto the client. My area of work as a Clinical Psychologist has been to specialise in helping clients who have experienced trauma, and so these issues of what topics can "safely" be introduced is a key concern. When working with people who have experienced trauma, it may be really important to the assessment and/or the intervention to speak about certain things that may be potentially very distressing to the client. In these situations, their safety is always my first concern, as to inadvertently "trigger" a fight/flight or dissociation response by blundering into talking about something when the client is not ready could be quite harmful. So timing, working at the clients' pace, working within their window of tolerance and their threshold for managing to talk about distressing material is one of the key skills to learn.

I am happy to be able to share my research findings about the reflected speech device of "you said" with other professionals, as I think it helps us all in this process of working within the client's scope of tolerance. The result of doing so, in my mind, is to facilitate a sense of safety and control for the client that is fundamental to any trauma work. Of course, it may be that the client has something important or difficult to share that they have not mentioned before, and so in these situations, patience, sensitivity, and creating a safe environment are important in helping a client to find ways to initially speak about their distress. When that first mention is made about the thing that they find most painful and shaming in their life, they may quickly move on or change the subject for fear of judgment or fear of their own emotions in relation to that topic. However, if it has at some time actually been uttered, it is now within the shared space of knowledge that the professional and the client hold together. It is a precious thing that the client has found a way to share that difficult and painful thing with another human being.

"You said" reflected speech gives an opportunity to carefully re-introduce a topic when a distraction, avoidance, or subject change has shifted the conversation away from that area. It is also an *invitational* approach that proposes back to the client the thing they have said and offers them an opportunity to elaborate further if they feel that they can. This invitation is important when working with hurting people who have experienced trauma, abuse, and shame, which often by their very nature have been ruthlessly imposed upon them against their choice or will. Invitational language like this is much more respectful of clients and honours the courage they draw upon to look for and receive help form others. It is also an approach that may be more appropriate within certain cultural contexts where propositional or invitational and collaborative ways of talking are more culturally acceptable. Within professional contexts a common phrase for this kind of approach might be "client-centred" language, which is a way of conversing that honours the journey of the client, and the need to progress in their own way at their own pace. At the same time, it provides an opportunity to explore important areas such as risk a little further, which is often our professional responsibility. As shown in extract three in this chapter, "you said" can be used effectively to explore risk by using reflected speech as a platform to ask for a little more detail or information about the statement provided that indicated a potential risk concern.

As a clinical academic, it has been fascinating to be involved in this research project and to look at naturally occurring data to examine real-world conversational practices within an institutional setting. From a professional point of view, it is an excellent process of reflective practice to watch these videos and to look at transcripts of mental health professionals engaged in their work. This kind of reflection using practice-based data is an excellent way to further develop good practice, and as the research has shown, to tease out the intricacies of *how* we go about our work within helping professions through the language that we use. Although anecdotally through my own clinical work and observation of colleagues and students, I could see that using reflected speech was an integral part of our work, it is only through engaging in a rigorous research process that the nuggets of information about how it operates were revealed.

Concluding comments

Reflected speech shares some linguistically similar features to reported speech, such as re-introducing a previously discussed topic into the current conversational interaction. However, in reflected speech, rather than reported on what someone else has said, the speaker reflects back the words of the addressee. In effect rather than using the canonical "he said/she said", the speaker would use the preface "you said". This preface has been shown to be part of a sequence of interactional turns established between the two speakers wherein the topic being introduced using reflected speech is established as an accepted basis for proceeding. In a clinical setting, it can be used effectively as part of the assessment or therapy stage, especially where sensitive topics such as those related to risk assessment are important to raise. It can also assist the therapeutic process between adult therapist and young client, by reducing the power imbalance and by invitation as to which topics of conversation are made immediately relevant.

The chapter has drawn on some of my own research into this discursive device to show the value of re-introducing a topic that a child or young person had previously mentioned. It both allows the professional some scope to select or have influence over which topic is made currently relevant, whilst simultaneously demonstrating an acknowledgement that it was the child or young person's topic in the first instance. Three functional outcomes of the use of reflected speech were demonstrated and discussed which were: to re-introduce a topic, to provide a platform for a follow-up question, and to elicit elaboration and/or clarification.

The chapter has also provided some thoughts about how knowledge of this discursive resource may help professionals to collaboratively and

Table 4.1 An abridged glossary of the transcription symbols used in conversation analysis

Symbol	Description
(.)	A micropause – too short to time
(0.7)	A timed pause
[ ]	Square brackets show where speech overlaps
> <	A faster pace of speech
< >	A slower pace of speech
Underline	Denotes a raise in volume or emphasis
↑	Rise in intonation
↓	Drop in intonation
CAPITALS	Louder or shouted words
(h)	Laughter
=	Latching – where the end of one sentence is immediately connected to the next line where the same symbol is seen
:::	A stretched sound

dynamically establish agreed topics to discuss during a session. This is especially relevant in relation to the topic of risk and other potentially embarrassing or sensitive topics that might be difficult for the child or young person to raise. The details of how one might use the turn-by-turn sequence of reflected speech in clinical practice have been explained carefully, by referring back to the detailed data extracts used in the chapter. The value of using recordings of naturally occurring institutional conversations as a tool for reflective practice, has been highlighted as a way to identify areas of good practice. As a Clinical Psychologist, the practical applications of using this strategy have been explored in the reflective practice section, and the implications for clinical practice considered.

Note

1 A glossary of transcription symbols is provided in Table 4.1 at the end of the chapter for reference.

References

Antaki, C., 2007. Mental-health practitioners' use of idiomatic expressions in summarizing client's accounts. *J. Pragmat. 39*, 527–541.

Antaki, C., O'Reilly, M., 2014. Either/or questions in psychiatric assessments: The effect of the seriousness and order of the alternatives. *Discourse Stud. 16* (3), 327–345.

Bone, C., O'Reilly, M., Karim, K., Vostanis, P., 2014. 'They're not witches …': Young children and their parents' perceptions and experiences of Child and Adolescent Mental Health Services. *Child: Care, Health Dev. 41* (3), 450–458.

Chu, B., Kendall, P., 2004. Positive associations of child involvement and treatment outcome within a manual-based cognitive behavioral treatment with anxiety. *J. Consulting Clin. Psychol. 72*, 821–829.

Drew, P., Chatwin, J., Collins, S., 2001. Conversation analysis: A method for research into interactions between patients and health-care professionals. *Health Expectations 4* (1), 58–70.

Heritage, J., 1984. A change-of-state token and aspects of its sequential placement. In: Atkinson, J.M., Heritage, J. (Eds.), *Structures of Social Action: Studies in Conversation Analysis*. Cambridge University Press, Cambridge, pp. 299–345.

Holt, E., 1996. Reporting on talk: The use of direct reported speech in conversation. *Res. Lang. Soc. Interact. 29*, 219–245.

Hutchby, I., 2002. Resisting the incitement to talk in child counselling: Aspects of the utterance "I don't know". *Discourse Stud. 4* (2), 147–168.

Hutchby, I., Wooffitt, R., 1999. *Conversation Analysis: Principles, Practices and Applications*. Cambridge UK: Polity Press.

Jefferson, G., 2004. Glossary of transcript symbols with an introduction. In: Lerner, G.H. (Ed.), *Conversation Analysis: Studies from the First Generation*. John Benjamins, Amsterdam, pp. 13–31.

Kiyimba, N., O'Reilly, M., 2018. Reflecting on what "you said" as a way of re-introducing difficult topics in child mental health assessments. *Child. Adolesc. Ment. Health 23* (3), 148–154.

Kiyimba, N., Lester, J., O'Reilly, M., 2019. *Using Naturally Occurring Data in Qualitative Health Research: A Practical Guide*. Springer, London.

MacMartin, C., 2008. Resisting optimistic questions in narrative and solution-focused therapies. In: Peräkylä, A., Antaki, C., Vehviläinen, S., Leudar, I. (Eds.), *Conversation Analysis and Psychotherapy*. Cambridge University Press, Cambridge, pp. 80–99.

McCabe, R., Heath, C., Burns, T., Priebe, S., 2002. Engagement of patients with psychosis in the consultation: Conversation analytic study. *BMJ 325*, 1148–1151.

O'Reilly, M., Karim, K., Kiyimba, N., 2015. Question use in child mental health assessments and the challenges of listening to families. *BJPsych Open 1* (2), 116–120.

O'Reilly, M., Kiyimba, N., Lester, J., Muskett, T., 2020. Reflective interventionist conversation *analysis. Discourse & Communication 14* (6), 619–634.

Parker, N., 2003. *A Discursive Analysis of Family Therapy Interactions*. Unpublished PhD Thesis. Loughborough University, Loughborough, UK.

Parker, N., O'Reilly, M., 2013. Reflections from behind the screen: Avoiding therapeutic rupture when utilising reflecting teams. *Family Journal: Counseling Couples Families 21* (2), 170–179.

Parkin, A., Frake, C., Davison, I., 2003. A triage clinic in a Child and Adolescent Mental Health Service. *Child. Adolesc. Ment. Health 8* (4), 177–183.

Peräkylä, A., 2013. Conversation analysis in psychotherapy. In: Sidnell, J., Stivers, T. (Eds.), *The Handbook of Conversation Analysis*. Wiley-Blackwell, Chichester, pp. 551–574.

Potter, J., 2002. Two kinds of natural. *Discourse Stud. 4* (4), 539–542.

Sacks, H., Schegloff, E.A., Jefferson, G., 1978. A simplest systematics for the organization of turn taking for conversation. *In Studies in the Organization of Conversational Interaction*. Academic Press, pp. 7–55.

Stivers, T., 2001. Negotiating who presents the problem: Next speaker selection in pediatric encounters. *J of Comm. 51*(2), 252–282.

Voutilainen, L., Peräkylä, A., Ruusuvuori, J., 2010. Misalignment as a therapeutic resource. *Qualitative Res. Psychol.* 7 (4), 299–315.

Weatherall, A., Gibson, M., 2015. "I'm going to ask you a very strange question": A conversation analytic case study of the miracle technique in solution-based therapy. *Qualitative Res. Psychol.* 12 (2), 162–181.

White, A., 2003. *Womens' Usage of Specific Linguistic Functions in the Context of Casual Conversation: Analysis and Discussion.* Dissertation. University of Birmingham, Birmingham, U.K.

Ziolkowska, J., 2009. Positions in doctors' questions during psychiatric interviews. *Qualitative Health Res.* 19 (11), 1621–1631.

Chapter 5

Children's communication and their mental health

Perspectives from speech and language therapy

Judy Clegg

Introduction

Children and young people with social, emotional, and mental health difficulties (SEMH) often have communication difficulties. These communication difficulties are usually not identified. Therefore, their vulnerability increases as they are unable to access and engage in support and services available to them (Cross et al., 2001; Clegg, 2020). The speech and language therapy profession works with these children and young people to meet their communication needs. This chapter will discuss how practitioners across health, education, and social services can identify and understand communication difficulties and how to support these needs to enable more effective communication. Ultimately, this will promote the psycho-social adjustment and outcomes for the most vulnerable children and young people in our society.

Understanding children's communication development

Communication is essential to our practice when working with vulnerable children and young people. We expect them to listen to and understand us, carry out our instructions, share their experiences with us, read information, discuss complex concepts with us, correctly interpret our communicative behaviours, and communicate with us in a socially appropriate way. We take communication for granted because we assume our children and young people can communicate effectively. However, research shows many vulnerable children and young people have developmental communication difficulties we do not account for in our interactions with them (Anderson, Hawes, and Snow, 2016; Gilmour, Hill, and Place, 2004; Sylvestre and Merette, 2010).

Communication is complex and children learn to be competent communicators at a very young age. The first 5 years is a rapid period of speech, language, and communication development. Infants learn to clearly say the sounds of the language(s) they are exposed to. They learn words and their meanings as well as the grammatical system of a language. They become adept at putting words and grammatical structures together into meaningful phrases, sentences, and narratives. They use their developing speech and language to communicate with others in a meaningful and socially and culturally acceptable way.

By school age, most children are competent communicators (see Figure 5.1). Speech and language are essential precursors to learning to read and write. Children need to know the sounds of their language(s) and how this maps on to letters as well as knowing the meanings of words and how these relate to the written word. Competence in spoken language is needed before learning to read and write. Speech, language, and communication continues to develop through adolescence and into adult life (see Figure 5.2) (see Drewett this volume for discussion of adult settings). Communication development continues into adolescence with the acquisition of higher-level skills such as learning specific and abstract school curriculum words. At this age, learning is primarily through reading rather than spoken language. If language and then literacy is not secure, learning becomes even more compromised at this stage with significant consequences for educational achievement. Children learn to communicate with their peers in socially and culturally acceptable ways which usually differs from how they communicate with their families and professionals in their educational contexts.

By school age, most children are competent communicators and can:

❖ **Speak clearly:** they have learnt the sounds of the language(s) they are learning and say most of these sounds in words clearly. Some children may find some of the harder speech sounds difficult to say such as the 'y' sound in 'yellow'.

❖ **Understand instructions:** they listen to and understand short verbal instructions. Children will still rely on contextual cues to help their understanding such as real examples of objects, pictures, and people.

❖ **Know sounds and start to match these to letters:** they start to understand a sound they say in a word matches a symbol, i.e., a written letter. This is an early stage of literacy.

❖ **Say an enormous range of vocabulary:** they have 1000s of words they understand and say. These are concrete words where the meaning of the word is obvious as well as harder to learn abstract words, e.g., words we use to describe feelings.

❖ **Use a grammatical system in their talking:** they say complex sentences such as 'it's fish and chips today because it is a Friday and not Monday'. They put these sentences together into accounts, explanations, and narratives.

❖ **Use a wide range of communicative functions:** they use their speech and language to argue, explain, describe, negotiate, narrate, request information, and many other functions.

❖ **Communicate using verbal and non-verbal means:** children are becoming competent in managing conversations using eye-contact, taking turns, and other non-verbal means.

Figure 5.1 A summary of the communication skills achieved by children aged 4 to 5 years.

By the end of adolescence, most young people can:

❖ **Follow and understand complex instructions:** they understand long instructions with abstract information which does not follow the word order of the sentence e.g., 'Before you collect your information, complete the form and give it to the receptionist'.

❖ **Follow and understand abstract instruction words:** they understand words such as evaluate, compile, understand, reflect, analyse and phrases such as find themes, highlight the challenges. For example, if you **reflect** on your behaviour this morning, what do you think you could have done differently?

❖ **Give long and complex narratives:** they ensure the listener understands their long account or explanation. They check with the listener to make sure he/she is following. They know when to clarify and re-phrase.

❖ **Talk in long sentences (with more than 12 words):** they engage in in-depth discussions and conversations without needing prompting.

❖ **Understand emotions and how to identify and communicate these:** they identify their feelings and explain these to others. They use communication to understand how to manage difficult feelings and emotions.

❖ **Able to switch easily between informal and formal styles of talking depending on the audience:** they communicate appropriately with different listeners and audiences. They can change their communication style to do this. Young people who are multi-lingual can adapt their communication style to fit the different socio-cultural contexts they are growing up in.

❖ **Fully understand and use inferential language such as humour, sarcasm, metaphors, idioms and irony:** they know when someone is being sarcastic or using irony and they know how to respond to this appropriately.

❖ **Engage fully in written information:** they access and understand complex written information. They complete complex written tasks such as form filling, handling documents and completing online applications and learning.

Figure 5.2 A summary of the communication skills achieved by young people during adolescence.

There is much variation in these stages and so, the challenge in the early years is understanding which children are not developing as expected and will go on to have difficulties in their communication development. The pattern of communication development and the profile of communication difficulties in children with developmental disorders such as Autism Spectrum Disorder (ASD) and Down syndrome is well documented (Fidler and Daunhauer, 2011; Howlin and Charman, 2011). Other children may be delayed in their communication development and with early identification and support these communication difficulties can resolve. It is a challenge to accurately identify at a young age which children are delayed and whether this delay will resolve. A delay can be the first identifiable sign of persisting communication difficulties as part of a pervasive developmental disorder. Children who continue to experience difficulties in their communication development at age 5 years will continue to have persisting communication difficulties with implications for other aspects of their lives. These include their learning and educational progress, their friendships and relationships and their social, emotional, and behavioural development. Many children experience difficulties in their communication development and often there is no identifiable cause for this. These children are often the most challenging to identify and support.

The impact of persisting communication difficulties on a child's life is pervasive. Identifying this impact is challenging as it is not always obvious. Let's consider the impact of Amy's communication difficulties at 6 years and then at 14 years old.

The everyday impact of communication difficulties for Amy who is 6 years old

Amy entered a mainstream school over a year ago. Concerns about her communication development were raised when a Health Visitor noticed she was not talking at the age of 2 and a half. Amy is now talking but her speech is not clear and difficult for others to understand. Amy speaks in phrases rather than sentences and is not able to give detailed answers to questions, detailed descriptions, and accounts. Amy finds it hard to learn new words, so she does not have the range of vocabulary expected for her age. She finds it hard to process and understand what people say to her. In the classroom, as a result of her communication difficulties, Amy finds it harder than other children to:

Do what she is asked to do: Amy does not consistently follow the teacher's verbal instructions and she relies on following the other children to help her. Sometimes this is successful but often, she is left behind. She is reprimanded for this by the teaching staff.

Contribute and engage fully in activities: As Amy is not able to understand the language around her, she is not able to engage with her learning. Amy is not able to put her hand up and answer questions or complete the worksheets on time. Amy is always working harder than other children to understand what she is being asked to do.

Explain her actions, her thoughts, and her feelings to others: Amy does not have the communication abilities to tell others her thoughts and feelings. She has not learnt words that describe her feelings and so, others are not able to understand her experiences.

Communicate effectively to be able to make friends and establish relationships: Amy cannot navigate her complex social environment. The children and teaching staff do not consistently understand her and there are many times when she cannot communicate her needs to others. Amy is quiet and withdrawn, not wanting to join in with other children and occasionally she tells other children to "go away".

The school is aware of her speech difficulties as these are obvious to the staff and other children. However, her language difficulties are less obvious but are having a significant impact for her. Amy is behind with her learning and educational achievement at the end of primary school. Amy then makes the transition to a mainstream secondary school.

The everyday impact of communication difficulties for Amy who is now 14 years old

At age 14 years, Amy continues to need time and support to process and understand. Her speech is unclear to others. She does not have the words to communicate with others about her needs. She finds the complex world of adolescent social relationships very difficult. At 14 years, Amy is:

Struggling at school academically: Amy continues to find it hard to learn the words and concepts she needs in order to learn. She has literacy difficulties, which means she cannot engage in her learning and show her learning effectively.

Lonely and vulnerable: Amy has few friends and a limited social network. Others perceive her as different and so she is at risk of victimisation.

Low in confidence and self-esteem: Amy perceives herself as different to her peers. She struggles with her schoolwork and knows she is failing.

Unable to access effective support: Amy must work harder than others to access support, e.g., reading resources aimed to support young people as these are always written and not accessible to her.

Invisible: Amy's communication difficulties are invisible to others. Amy is good at "masking" where she pretends to understand by working hard to use the context to help her. Therefore, teachers and others are not aware of how much she is struggling. Amy is often perceived as passive, dis-interested, not engaged, not compliant, and at times defiant.

Most children are competent communicators when they start formal schooling. Children continue in their communication development into adolescence and adult life. For some children, their communication does not develop as expected. Sometimes there is an identifiable cause for this and a clear profile of the subsequent and persisting communication difficulties. Often, there is no clear cause and these children continue with a profile of persisting communication difficulties which impacts on many aspects of their lives.

Identifying communication difficulties in vulnerable children and young people

My own research and practice focus on understanding what happens to children and young people with persisting communication difficulties. We now know children and young people with persisting communication difficulties experience significant psycho-social difficulties. Much of this research focused on children and young people with a clinical diagnosis of Developmental Language Disorder (DLD). This is a label that refers to children who experience significant difficulties in their communication development which is not easily explained by other cognitive or developmental difficulties. DLD co-occurs with many other developmental difficulties including SEMH difficulties. Years ago, I met and assessed adults with DLD in their 20s and 30s as well as those in the process of leaving formal education. We also interviewed them along with their parents and carers to find out more about their experiences and lives and what support and provision is needed. Our findings showed these children experienced many negative psycho-social outcomes including educational disengagement, lower-than-expected educational attainment, few friendships and relationships, bullying and victimisation, mental health difficulties including psychoses, securing and maintaining employment, and limited independent living. These psycho-social outcomes were unexpected and confirm that persisting communication difficulties increase the risk of negative psycho-social outcomes and life chances. The identification of mental health difficulties led to further research and practice with other vulnerable groups of children and young people. These are young people in the youth justice system, children and young people with adverse childhood experiences such as abuse and neglect, children and young people excluded from school as well as those with SEMH difficulties. The ultimate aim being to understand the role of communicative competence and communication difficulties in these children's life chances.

Our research (summarised in Clegg 2018, 2020) provides evidence to support an association between children's communication difficulties and their social, emotional, and mental health (SEMH). We know that over 50% of young people in the youth justice system have communication difficulties. Children excluded from mainstream schools because their behaviour is disruptive and challenging often have communication difficulties as do children and young people with SEMH and those in receipt of Child and Adolescent Mental Health Services (CAMHS) services. Our more recent research shows young people coming out of looked after provision also have communication difficulties (Clegg et al., 2019). Importantly, the communication difficulties in all these vulnerable populations have not previously been identified. It seems the other needs the child and/or young person presents with, often SEMH and challenging behaviour is the primary area of concern.

The failure to identify these communication difficulties earlier is interesting. Earlier, I discussed how often there are no identifiable cause(s) to explain why some children's communication does not develop as expected and children continue to have persisting communication difficulties. We know that a high proportion of children who grow up experiencing adverse childhood experiences (ACE) are likely to have communication difficulties. There are complex associations operating here such as home environments that do not adequately foster language learning, adverse and traumatic life events that negatively impact on children's development including their communication development, environments where children experience multiple care givers disrupting their attachment, and again impacting negatively on their development including their communication development (summarised in Clegg 2018, 2020). Communication difficulties may not be identified as other needs are more obvious and apparent, and therefore take priority, such as social, emotional, and behavioural difficulties. These children's communication difficulties may also not meet threshold for a clinical diagnosis such as DLD due to being associated with their other developmental needs, not being referred to speech and language therapy services, and perhaps even an unconscious but lowered expectation about the communicative competence of these children and young people.

Profiles of communication difficulties

Profiles of communication difficulties specific to diagnoses of SEMH are unlikely to be established due to the heterogeneity of children and young people with these diagnoses. Research to date has identified patterns of communication difficulties and related behaviours which are useful for practitioners to consider in our practice. The communication profiles of children with SEMH difficulties, specifically selective mutism, attention deficit hyperactivity disorder (ADHD), and attachment disorders are now examined. These disorders are chosen as there is some evidence to support associated communication profiles (Oerbeck et al., 2014; Sadiq et al., 2012; Walsh et al., 2014).

Selective mutism

Selective mutism, where children are unable to communicate verbally and sometimes non-verbally in certain situations, often school but communicate freely and as usual in other situations is now understood as an anxiety disorder or even a phobia. For reasons often not easily understood, a child develops a severe anxiety of talking and as a result, will stop talking in certain situations or contexts and with certain people. For some children, this resolves over time but for others it can be a persisting challenge with obvious implications for everyday aspects of their lives. By definition (see most recent diagnostic criteria in DSM-V), children with selective mutism do not usually present with previous existing communication difficulties. However, from the author's own experiences, selective mutism is often co-morbid with other developmental disorders such as ASD, learning disability and other SEMH. Speech difficulties also contribute to the anxiety children experience in talking thus making them more reluctant to talk. Reluctant talking can be a more friendly term to use, describing a broader range of children and young people who find talking anxiety provoking.

Attention deficit hyperactivity disorder (ADHD)

There is no one profile of communication difficulties specific to ADHD and instead children with ADHD can present with a broad range of difficulties across their speech, language, and communication. Often social communication is a focus as the behaviours intrinsic to ADHD such as inattention and impulsivity disrupt the children's social communication, e.g., not listening, interrupting others, and dominating conversations.

ADHD is highly comorbid with other developmental disorders and so it is likely that children with diagnoses of ADHD also have communication difficulties. These may be part of other developmental disorders such as ASD, learning difficulties, dyslexia, and SEMH. Where other developmental disorders are not present, children with ADHD may not be understanding because they are not able to attend and listen sufficiently to process the information they are hearing effectively. Taken together it is likely that children with ADHD do have difficulties understanding spoken language and other communication difficulties.

Attachment

Like ADHD, a range of communication difficulties has been identified in children with histories of disruptions in their attachment or with attachment disorders. Children with histories of significant abuse and neglect are reported to have high rates of communication difficulties. Therefore, disclosing their experiences will be challenging. These procedures rely on spoken communication and therefore modifications are needed to account for any communication difficulties.

Although profiles of communication difficulties are discussed in relation to diagnoses of SEMH, in reality, children present with complex profiles. Therefore, it is difficult to tease out specific profiles of communication difficulties associated with different SEMH difficulties. Furthermore, comorbidity is often high and differentiating the potential cause of communication difficulties becomes even more challenging. In reality and from the authors' own clinical experiences, issues around identifying profiles and causation is not always the priority. It is more important to identify a child's communication difficulties and how best to support these to enable the most effective communication. Families and professionals should consider the possibility of unidentified communication difficulties in children with SEMH to ensure these children are able to access and engage in the interventions offered to them.

Working with vulnerable children and young people with communication difficulties

A high proportion of vulnerable children and young people have persisting communication difficulties which are not routinely identified. The profession of speech and language therapy advocates the involvement of speech and language therapists to accurately assess their communication needs and to provide evidence-based interventions to facilitate more effective communication. The ultimate aim is to facilitate the child's or young person's communicative competence and his/her communicative environment to enable more effective engagement with education, health and social services to ensure optional psycho-social adjustment and outcomes. This aim is encapsulated in the five good standards of communication for children and young people with SEMH published by the RCSLT (Table 5.1).

The evidence base supporting the effectiveness of speech and language therapy (SLT) or communication interventions in this population is at an early stage. Case study research shows communication interventions can be effective in enabling children and young people with SEMH to learn

Table 5.1 Good standards of communication

Five Good Standards of Communication to be implemented for children and young people with SEMH

For those delivering the standards:	For those receiving the standards:
Standard 1: There is a detailed description of how best to communicate with individuals.	**Standard 1:** There is good information that tells people how best to communicate with me.
Standard 2: Services demonstrate how they support individuals to be involved with decisions.	**Standard 2:** Staff help me to be involved in making decisions about my care and support.
Standard 3: Staff value and use competently the best approaches to communication with each individual they support.	**Standard 3:** Staff are good at supporting me with my communication.
Standard 4: Services create opportunities, relationships, and environments that make individuals want to communicate.	**Standard 4:** I have lots of chances to communicate.
Standard 5: Individuals are supported to understand and express their needs in relation to their health and well-being.	**Standard 5:** Staff help me to understand and communicate about my health.
Cue the child or young person into what you are going to talk about	

language and so facilitate their engagement in their learning, as well as increasing their access to other interventions such as CAMHS and youth justice services (Clegg, 2014; Cross et al., 2001; Heneker, 2005). The interventions often take more time to implement due to the challenging needs of the children and young people. Training practitioners who work with children and young people to identify communication difficulties and to learn to use strategies to support these difficulties is also advocated. The communication interventions do not have to be implemented by speech and language therapists and a range of practitioners can learn to implement these interventions successfully. Indeed, a more cost-effective model of delivering communication interventions is for speech and language therapists to train practitioners in how to identify communication difficulties and to learn to implement strategies to facilitate communication across all the children and young people they work with. The developing evidence base is promising in showing the effectiveness of communication interventions in promoting more effective access and engagement (Bryan et al., 2015). Box 5.1 details practical tips we can employ to help us identify communication difficulties.

We know that communication difficulties make it harder for children and young people to engage and interact, to develop and to learn. If the approaches used by practitioners cannot accommodate these communication difficulties, then the children and young people will not be able to engage and interact and to develop and learn from these approaches. Box 5.2 shows the strategies we can use to help us modify our own communication to enable children and young people to communicate with us more effectively.

Finally, we can all modify the environment we work in to make it more communication friendly for our children and young people. Box 5.3 shows how we can make our environments more communication friendly.

A teenager with complex needs: Perspectives from speech and language therapy

I recently worked with a city council service, that supports young people in their transition from care to independence. These young people are between the ages of 16 and 25 years and have been in looked after provision, often experiencing multiple placements in foster and residential homes. Many of these very vulnerable young people have experienced multiple adverse childhood experiences and continue to experience significant challenges in many areas of their lives. The service was starting to recognise that communicating with many of their young people is challenging, citing issues around their engagement, interaction, compliance, and behaviour as well as mental health difficulties. Given their adverse childhood experiences and the high prevalence of developmental disorders, educational disengagement, and mental health difficulties reported in looked after children and young people, I considered it very likely that many of these young people would

---

Box 5.1   Practical tips for being alert

Six practical tips for being alert to communication difficulties

- **Assume there are communication difficulties:** consider communication across listening, understanding, talking, reading, writing, behaviour, and social communication.
- **Comorbidity of communication difficulties:** if the individual has other needs then it is very likely the individual also has communication difficulties.
- **Communication difficulties are hidden:** individuals often learn to pretend they are following and understanding and they are unlikely to say they are not understanding.
- **Behaviour is communication:** can the individual's behaviour be explained by communication difficulties, e.g., a child who seems disinterested and disengaged but is struggling to know what he is being asked to do.
- **Analyse communication:** think about the individual's communication. Is their speech clear? What sorts of words do they use? Do they use the same words repetitively or do they have lots of different words? Can they give you lots of details? Do they use lots of hesitations and filler type words such as "erm", "thing", "you know what I mean"? Do you have to keep asking questions or prompting the child or young person to try and get them to communicate with you? Is it hard work to engage the child or young person? Do they come across as rude as they do not communicate in the way expected of them? Refer to the communicative competence expected of children and young people in Figures 5.1 and 5.2. Are your expectations of the communicative competence of the children and young people you work with appropriate? Make sure your expectations are not too low and therefore you are not identifying potential difficulties.
- **Refer children and young people to speech and language therapy (SLT) services:** speech and language therapists are experts in communication. They work with vulnerable children and young people to identify their communication difficulties and to facilitate their communication as well as the communication environment to enable their access. They are not about speech and elocution.

---

have communication difficulties which were not identified and these would be impacting on their engagement with the service. Together, we worked to understand if these young people do have communication difficulties, the

---

Box 5.2   Practical tips for improving communication

Ten practical tips for improving practitioner's own communication

- **Talk slowly:** talk more slowly than you think is needed and pause between sentences.
- **Talk clearly:** you may need to increase the volume of your talking; try and reduce any background noise.
- **Highlight important words:** say the important words more loudly and clearly than the other words, e.g., We are **meeting** at **2 o'clock** on **Monday.**
- **Give time to process, think, and reply:** after asking a question or giving an instruction, wait for 5 seconds to give the individual time to process and understand. It will feel a long time to you but not to the individual. If there is no reply, then repeat what you have said, perhaps in a different easier way.
- **Cue the child or young person into what you are going to talk about:** tell the individual the plan, e.g., "First, we are going to talk about your Mum". "We've finished talking about Mum, now we will talk about school". "We've finished talking about school. Let's talk about going home". This structure helps the individual to focus and to know what is coming next.
- **Only use short sentences:** break long sentences up in to phrases and say these slowly with pauses in between them.
- **Use less words:** reduce the number of words you use.
- **Use more concrete words:** use easy-to-understand words.
- **Never use irony, sarcasm, and humour:** this is complex language which is hard to understand and easy to misinterpret.
- **Repeat key pieces of information:** this is useful to individuals and not patronising or irritating.
- **Use visual support:** use drawings, pictures, symbols, planners, and mind maps to support your talking.

---

nature of these, and how they could be supported by the service. Below is a case study from this work.

The key worker who worked with Rania described her as "volatile" and "difficult to engage" often not carrying out agreed actions from their meetings. At other times, she could be passive and emotional. Rania was 17 years old at the time of my involvement. Rania had entered care aged 6 years and was starting the process of making the transition away from care. She was living in her fourth placement and at the time was very keen to move to live independently. Rania had attended mainstream schools and college.

Box 5.3 Practical tips for environment

Six practical tips for creating communication-friendly environments

- **Show who and what you are:** make easily available photos of staff and key areas, rooms, equipment, and resources; explain roles in concrete terms, e.g., the term "Sarah is your key worker" can be simplified as "Sarah will help you". Take time to listen and build trust by spending time together engaging in everyday activities. Building trust can be key for a young person to feel confident in communicating with someone.
- **Make written information accessible:** any writing a child or young person is expected to read needs to be accessible.
- **Reduce information overload:** reduce the amount of written information in the environment; consider how overwhelming the amount of leaflets and posters in a waiting area may be.
- **Teach the words needed:** each context has its own terminology; identify the terms and words the child and young person needs to know to engage. For example, make sure the individual knows what is meant by the terminology staff use all the time such as "care pathway", "medication", "session", "occupational therapy", "counselling", "appointment", "therapy", "patient". Teach the child or young person these words and what these mean.
- **Make the environment visual:** try not to rely on talking as the main form of communication; use photographs, drawings, visual timetables, mind maps, symbols.
- **Use gestures:** try to use natural gesture in your talking, e.g., point to what you are talking about. Start to use some simple signs such as Makaton to support your talking.

Rania had not received any additional support for educational needs at school or college. Rania was starting an apprenticeship scheme and through this her reading and writing had been identified as a potential area of concern and so at the time of my involvement she was awaiting a dyslexia assessment. This was the first time literacy difficulties had been highlighted for Rania. Rania's first contact with mental health services had been at 11 years with diagnoses of depression and anxiety currently recorded. Rania was continuing to receive support from mental health services.

My involvement as a SLT was to profile Rania's communication. I spent time with Rania in various contexts including meetings with her key workers, interacting with others at service events, talking to Rania about her experiences to date and in meetings about the apprenticeship scheme she was starting to participate in.

From these contexts, I concluded the following:

- **Rania was not understanding fully when others were talking to her:** Rania appeared to listen but would not follow through on what she was asked to do such as contacting practitioners and completing forms to access support available to her. Rania always asked lots of questions about the content covered in meetings. As this happened at the end of meetings, there was not always enough time for the key worker to answer these questions. Rania often did not attend pre-arranged meetings or appointments including with her key workers but also with external agencies.
- **Rania was not able to access the plethora of verbal and written information given to her:** Rania was given a lot of written information to read and she was not able to read this to sufficiently understand what she needed to do to engage. Rania appeared overwhelmed by this.
- **Rania was angry and frustrated.** She was often upset at the start of meetings or came into the service centre very anxious, upset and sometimes angry. At these times, she wanted to see her keyworker and became upset when the relevant staff were not available. Rania did not seem to be able to follow the expected way of contacting her key worker.
- **Rania was hard to engage:** Rania often gave up. She would start an activity saying that it was "rubbish". Even with encouragement and support, she would not re-engage.
- **Rania was not able to talk about her feelings:** Rania would talk about being "fed up" or "bored" but she did not have other words to describe and communicate the very difficult emotions she was clearly feeling. Although Rania had a wide network of social contacts, she did not consider she had a strong support network.

As a qualified SLT, I was able to use standardised communication and literacy assessments to further understand Rania's difficulties. Rania and her key worker also completed a standardised report assessment where Rania rated her own communication skills. Her key worker also completed this same assessment but from his/her perspective as key worker. Similarities and differences in their perspectives were then compared. Rania had significant difficulties in her language and communication abilities as well as her literacy. Her scores were very low within the impairment range on all the assessments. The assessments confirmed significant difficulties in her understanding of spoken language, her ability to communicate effectively using language, and her vocabulary. Interestingly, her key worker rated her communication skills lower than Rania rated herself. Rania had awareness of areas she found difficult, these were her social communication, e.g., she was aware she did not understand others, that she was not able to follow what she needed to do and what others were asking of her, that she found relationships and friendships difficulties and was not able to express herself as she wanted to. Her key worker and Rania agreed Rania had more difficulties in her social communication than her language skills even though the standardised language assessments confirmed many difficulties in her language.

The next stage focused on working with Rania and her keyworker to address these needs. The aim was never to "solve" Rania's communication difficulties, instead for Rania to be able to access and engage more effectively with the support available to her. This involved working with Rania but perhaps more importantly working with her communication environment to make this more accessible. We did this collaboratively by:

- Devising a communication **profile:** This was a one-page easy-to-read summary explaining Rania's communication difficulties and strategies that help Rania. This was freely available to Rania and all staff to read and use. All staff were able to easily and quickly know that Rania has communication difficulties and strategies to use to support these.
- Implementing **visual support:** Staff learnt to support their talking with pictures, symbols, drawings, and writing of single key words. Visual timetables were key here. This was a way of showing Rania through drawing and simple words, the plan of each activity/interaction. When each activity was completed this was marked. Rania could see what she was being asked to do and knew how she was progressing so she knew when the activity would end. A timer was helpful here too, so a 30-minute session could easily be "seen" by Rania and she knew how much longer she needed to focus for.
- Using **accessible communication** at all times: The visual support above was adopted into all interactions and activities with Rania. This included written information too. A valuable tool was the development (in collaboration with Rania) of a visual diagram of her escalation of emotions and the strategies to use at each stage to help her manage these emotions. Staff learned how to simplify their language and to slow down, giving her more time to process and respond.
- Developing a **vocabulary of emotions:** In collaboration with Rania, a set of ten emotion words most relevant to Rania were identified. Rania learnt these words in terms of recognising the feelings these words mapped on to for her. These were made accessible (as per points above) and a visual dictionary of these feelings devised. Rania and staff used these in all their interactions. This enabled Rania to communicate when she felt unable to do something and asking for help rather than reverting to her learnt destructive pattern of behaviours.
- Learning to **self-monitor** her communication: Rania learnt how to say when she was not understanding and to ask for support.

Reflections

Over time, Rania became more engaged with two key members of staff and she was able to participate more fully in the interventions offered to her. I learnt how to work with a group of professionals I had not worked with before. I was struck by how skilled all the staff were in working with very vulnerable young people. I was very surprised by the under-identification of communication difficulties in this population. Rania very likely had these communication difficulties from a very young age, but it was only at the age of 17 years that her dyslexia difficulties were first highlighted which then led to concerns about her communication. Some of the young people I worked with had very late diagnoses of developmental disorders such ASD, learning difficulties, and even hearing impairments. I presume this late identification was due to the focus being more on behaviour without always thinking of difficulties that may underlie behaviour. The late identification of communication difficulties in Rania and others means that young people are struggling with these difficulties which then impact on other aspects of their lives. For many others, these communication difficulties are not identified.

It was a lengthy process and challenging to engage all staff. Rightly, some staff felt using this approach and strategies was in some way "patronising" and "childlike" for Rania. It is always a challenge to implement this approach in an age-appropriate way, particularly when using drawings and pictures. I appreciated this viewpoint, and in the future, taking the time to find more age appropriate resources will be valuable.

I am mindful these young people have many complex issues, and communicative competence and communication difficulties are only one aspect of this. I reflected their challenges will never be resolved by looking more closely at their communicative competence and supporting their communicative needs. However, ensuring more effective ways of communicating and making communication accessible has clear benefits in enabling young people to engage and participate to their full potential in the support and provision offered to them.

Conclusions

Practitioners need to be alert to communication difficulties in vulnerable children and young people. Identifying and supporting communication difficulties will facilitate engagement in the interventions aimed to support them. Identifying communication difficulties, improving our own communication, and creating communication friendly environments will increase engagement and ultimately lead to facilitating the life chances of our most vulnerable children and young people.

References

Anderson, S., Hawes, D., Snow, P., 2016. Language impairments among youth offenders: A systematic review. *Child. Youth Serv. Rev. 65*, 195–203.

Bryan, K., Garvani, G., Gregory, J., Kilner, K., 2015. Language difficulties and criminal justice: The need for earlier intervention. *Int. J. Lang. Commun. Disord. 50* (6), 763–775.

Clegg, J., 2014. Curriculum vocabulary learning intervention for children with social, emotional and behavioural difficulties (SEBD): Findings from a case study series. *Emotional Behavioural Difficulties 19* (1), 106–127.

Clegg, J., 2018. Teenagers' communication and their mental health. In: Spencer, S. (Ed.), *Supporting Adolescents with Language Disorders*. J&R Press, Guildford, UK.

Clegg, J., 2020. Children's communication and their mental health. In: Walsh, I., Jagoe, C. (Eds.), *Communication and Mental Health Disorders: Developing Theory, Growing Practice*. J&R Press, Daventry, UK.

Clegg, J., Crawford, E., Mathews, D., Spencer, S., 2019. Identifying and supporting the language and communication needs of care leavers to maximise their transition from care to independence. *Child Language Symposium*, July 10–12 2019, University of Sheffield, UK.

Cross, M., Blake, P., Tunbrige, N., Gill, T., 2001. Collaborative working to promote the communication skills of a 14-year-old student with emotional, behavioural, learning and language difficulties. *Child. Lang. Teach. Ther. 17*, 227–246.

Fidler, D., Daunhauer, L., 2011. Down Syndrome: General overview. In: Howlin, P., Charman, T., Ghaziuddin, M. (Eds.), *The SAGE Handbook of Developmental Disorders*. SAGE Publications Ltd, London, UK.

Gilmour, J., Hill, B., Place, M., Skuse, D.H., 2004. Social communication deficits in conduct disorder: A clinical and community survey. *J. Child. Psychol. Psychiatry 45*, 967–978.

Heneker, S., 2005. Speech and language therapy support for pupils with behavioural, emotional and social difficulties (BESD) – A pilot project. *Br. J. Spec. Educ. 32* (2), 86–91.

Howlin, P., Charman, T., 2011. Autism spectrum disorders: Interventions and outcome. In: Howlin, P., Charman, T., Ghaziuddin, M. (Eds.), *The SAGE Handbook of Developmental Disorders*. Sage Publications Ltd, London, UK.

Oerbeck, B., Stein, M., Wentzel-Larsen, T., Langsrud, O., Kristensen, H., 2014. A randomized controlled trial of a home and school-based intervention for selective mutism-defocused communication and behavioural techniques. *Child. Adolesc. Ment. Health 19* (3), 192–198.

Royal College of Speech and Language Therapists, 2019. Supporting children and young people with social, emotional and mental health needs (SEMH): The five good communication standards. https://www.rcslt.org/-/media/docs/Supporting-children-A4_No_Marks.pdf. (accessed 8 November 2020).

Sadiq, F., Slator, L., Law, J., Skuse, D., Gillberg, C., Minnis, H., 2012. A comparison of the pragmatic skills of children with reactive attachment disorder and high functioning autism. *Eur. Child. Adolesc. Psychiatry 21*, 267–276.

Aims of the chapter

Given the high numbers of children and young people with mental health difficulties who are self-harming, it is imperative that when engaging them in an assessment to determine if there is mental health need, a risk assessment for self-harm is also conducted. The focus for this chapter is on communication in initial mental health assessments in secondary care. However, it is important that practitioners in primary care are also aware of the prevalence and statistics around self-harm and suicidal behaviours in children and young people and be prepared and skilled to ask those kinds of questions. In this chapter, we examine how question design is important for engaging children and young people in these kinds of conversations and present good practice examples of how questions can be constructed to encourage interaction. These good practices are translatable from the mental health setting to broader communication techniques for practitioners working in other areas.

The research

Initial assessments are typically conducted to determine if a child or young person has a diagnosable mental health condition and/or if they meet the criteria for psychological or psychiatric intervention via specialist services or another appropriate agency. These first appointments are an important part of the process of screening for symptoms, identifying risk and providing an initial formulation of what the presenting difficulties might be (Mash and Hunsley, 2005). Typically, in these assessments, family members attend with the child or young person and collectively they present their concerns through a narrative of symptoms, behaviours, and feelings to a clinical practitioner or practitioners. This narrative provided by family members together with the questions asked by practitioners are an essential part of gathering important information to inform decision-making. A key component of this are the questions around risk of harm *to* and *from* others and risk of harm *to self* (see Reeves, this volume for further discussion).

The research study from which data are drawn to illustrate key messages in this chapter was one focused on initial mental health assessments in a secondary care CAMHS setting of children and young people in the UK. Following a rigorous ethical process within the NHS Research Ethics process, (i.e., National Research Ethics Service), approval to conduct the study was granted. A purposeful sample of all consenting first appointments (but excluding urgent referrals) were included and video recorded. Assessments were conducted by a multidisciplinary team of practitioners including consultant, staff-grade, and trainee psychiatrists, clinical and assistant psychologists, community psychiatric nurses (CPNs), occupational therapists, and psychotherapists. All 29 practitioners from the team participated.

Each assessment was approximately 90 minutes long and 28 families consented to be recorded. The children and young people ranged from 6–17 years old (mean age 11 years), and 64% were male and 36% were female. Children and young people attended with one or both parents (27 mothers, 8 fathers), and sometimes with siblings, extended family members, or other professionals.

The data collected were analysed qualitatively, following a detailed transcription system. The specific form of data analysis was a specialised technique called conversation analysis. Conversation analysis (CA) is an approach that focuses on language, that is, conversations that take place in real-world settings. The specific type of conversation analysis we used was Reflective Interventionist Conversation Analysis (RICA) which prioritises partnerships between academics and practitioners (O'Reilly et al., 2020). These conversations therefore occur naturally, and in analytic terms, conversation analysts call this naturally occurring data. This has the advantage of representing interactions as they occur in real life, rather than retrospective accounts that might be collected through interviews or focus groups (Kiyimba, Lester, and O'Reilly, 2019). We were particularly interested in this CAMHS setting in how healthcare practitioners asked questions and how effective those questions were in collecting assessment relevant information. In the examples we present in this chapter, the set of practices examined were question-answer sequences where practitioners focused on asking children and young people about self-harm and suicidal ideation. All extracts of data that included questions and answers about self-harm and suicidal ideation were collated to examine patterns and similarities/differences between them. This resulted in 27 sequences of talk for closer analytic scrutiny.

Importantly, collating *all* examples of these risk questions we identified that it was only in about half (15 of the 28) cases that practitioners specifically asked about self-harm and/or suicidal ideation (O'Reilly, Kiyimba, and Karim, 2016). This was an important finding that was valuable for the mental health team to reflect on in terms of their own processes for monitoring and developing good practice procedures. This is because it is globally recommended that any person over aged 10 years experiencing emotional distress would benefit from being asked about any thoughts or plans for self-harm or suicide (World Health Organization, 2016). This was a surprising finding, and speculatively or anecdotally there may be a range of reasons why they did not ask this question. While we do not have data to evidence these possible reasons, it may be that the case that the practitioners:

- Did not remember to do so
- Were not sure how to phrase such a question
- Felt awkward in the context of the specific assessment
- Were not confident what to do if the answer was yes
- Ran out of time to do so

- Thought the child might be too young for self-harm to be an issue to consider
- Made assumptions that if there was a likelihood of neurodevelopmental issues that the child would not be self-harming
- Had concerns that it may put ideas into the child's head
- Worry that it might upset the parents
- Kept the question for a second assessment appointment and the question was asked there (some families did not complete in one session).

As we are speculating here as to the possible reasons why the question was not asked, however, earlier work has suggested that professionals do feel some anxiety when working with clients with suicidal thoughts (Reeves, 2010; Reeves, this volume). We recommend that future research investigates the challenges of asking risk questions. In this chapter, our focus for communication can only be on the types of questions asked and their respective utility as this is the evidence available through the data.

Research findings

Whether you are in a position of needing to gather further information about these sensitive issues of self-harm and/or suicidal ideation or if you are responding to a child or young person who has volunteered information, it is helpful to think about how those questions and responses are phrased. This is in part because it will give you more confidence in how to handle those conversions and partly to help the child or young person to express what is going on and how they are feeling. The research findings from our project are presented in this chapter in such a way as to demonstrate some useful strategies for engaging in these conversations. We examine good practice examples of designing questions to assess for risk in ways that communicate effectively with children and young people about self-harm and suicidal ideation.

Asking risk assessment questions

As previously noted, in our data we illustrated that despite being a mental health setting where one may expect risk assessments to be routinely addressed, mental health professionals did not consistently ask about self-harm and suicide. Indeed, we highlighted earlier that only 15 of the 28 children and young people were engaged in these conversations during the initial assessment. The issue here is that if children and young people are not asked, they may not volunteer that information. The implications of this could potentially be quite serious if risk is not identified at an early enough stage. Thus, in presenting these guidelines on *how* to ask those questions, our hope is that practitioners working with children and young people will become more confident in doing so. Basically, our findings demonstrate that there are two core types of question design that seem to work well in encouraging children or young people to engage in dialogue about sensitive and emotional issues, like self-harm and suicidal ideation. First, is to gradually and incrementally build questions to lead up to more complex and challenging areas. Second, is to normalise or externalise the question as a procedural requirement.

Incremental building

An incremental questioning style is characterised by taking a gradual, step-by-step approach. Working incrementally, a person might start with something small and work up to something bigger; or may start with something easy and work up to something more difficult; or start from something general and work toward something specific. In conversation when working up to asking about something potentially sensitive or complex, the incremental approach is effective. The reason for this is because it starts gradually by asking general questions about feelings and works towards more specific questions about risk of harm to self, and eventually suicidal thoughts (see Yarn and Bromley, this volume, for a discussion of communicating feelings and depression). The benefit of this approach is that the risk question does not seem to "come out of nowhere". Furthermore, this incremental style of asking is more child-centred as it allows your later questions to be more responsive to their initial answers and is therefore more tailored to their specific situation.

The data example that follows is taken from our paper (O'Reilly et al., 2016, p. 483). This is quite a long example. To show the incremental steps that are built through the conversation we indicate where these steps are with arrows at certain junctures. In this example a Consultant Child and Adolescent Psychiatrist (referred to as Prac in the extract) is addressing a young person (referred to as YP in the extract) aged 13 years (taken from family 18 in the data). In terms of transcription symbols, where a word (or part word) is underlined, it means there was emphasis, and numbers in brackets denote time in seconds (0.91 seconds) – less than one second.

Extract 1:
```
1. Prac→   Is there any other way you show your frustration
2.         (0.91) you said you hit
3. YP      Yeah I h[it doors] hit doors
4. Prac            [doors]
5. YP      there's a massive hole in my door
6. Prac→   Yeah so you hit doors anything else?
7. YP      No
8. Prac→   Or hurting yourself?
9. YP      Yeah
10. Prac→  What d'you do?
11. YP     I slit my wrists once
```

```
12. Prac→  When was that?
13. YP     Erm (1.44) when we went doctors and they referred to
14.        CAMHS
15. Prac→  Is that a one-off thing or have you done it before?
16. YP     Er (0.32) done it a couple o' times
17. Prac   Couple of times is what's the purpose of doing that?
18. YP     I don't know I didn't want to hurt anyone an' just
19.        (0.35) it relieves it relieves the anger an' it just
20.        gets it away
21. Prac   So so relieves anger?
22.        (4.53)
23. Prac→  Is there an intention to kill yourself?
24. YP     I (0.31) like (0.39) stupid things like taking loads
25.        of paracetamol or som'ing (0.78) somfing like that
26. Prac→  Have you ever done that?
27. YP     Yeah
```

All of the incremental questions have been highlighted with an arrow (→) and we repeat them here in order as follows:

- Is there any other way you show your frustration (line 1)
- you hit doors anything else? (line 6)
- Or hurting yourself? (line 8)
- Whatd'you do? (line 10)
- When was that? (line 12)
- Is that a one-off thing or have you done it before? (line 15)
- what's the purpose of doing that? (line 17)
- Is there an intention to kill yourself? (line 23)
- Have you ever done that? (line 26)

When looking closely at this conversation, we can see that the psychiatrist starts this segment of the assessment with a general exploratory question about the young person's previous expression of feeling frustrated. By asking if there is "any other way" they can express this frustration, the psychiatrist is gently opening up the conversation to allow room for the young person to talk about risky behaviour if it was an issue. Notably, after a pause where there is no immediate response from the young person, the psychiatrist uses a tag "you said you hit" which is interrupted by the young person confirming that they *hit doors.* Beginning a statement with "you said" is itself a useful engagement technique, as it keeps the conversation child-centred (see Kiyimba, this volume; Kiyimba and O'Reilly, 2018).

The second incremental question, "hit doors, anything else?" then moves the conversation forward as hitting doors potentially may have a risk to self or a risk to others. In establishing that the young person does not hit anything else (e.g., other people), the third incremental question focuses on risk to self. The psychiatrist achieves this by softened question format "hurting yourself". Within three incremental questions the psychiatrist has been able to ask the young person directly about whether they engage in self-harm or not, which received an affirmation. By asking a direct closed question, the only response option the young person had was yes or no.

Having successfully established that the young person had engaged in self-harm, the task of the psychiatrist was to identify the severity of the behaviour and whether it may involve risk to life. The following three questions asked by the psychiatrist therefore related to the specifics of what the self-harming behaviour is (line 10), how recent the last episode was (line 12), and how often they engaged in that behaviour (line 15). Once this was formally established, the next increment was to pursue a line of questioning on suicidal thinking. Here we see a link between self-harm and suicide by working to identify the "purpose" of the self-harm. Potentially the self-harm may be an emotional regulation strategy used by the young person or potentially it could be a way of engaging in suicidal behaviours. For example, when a person takes paracetamol, this could be to treat a headache, could be to self-poison, or could be to end one's life and thus the *purpose* of taking those tablets is relevant and important to the conversation. Although the young person initially stated that the purpose was an emotional regulation strategy (*relieves the anger*) this would not necessarily preclude it also being used with an intention of ending their life. Therefore, the very specific clarification sought by the psychiatrist served to ensure that there was absolute clarity on the issue "is there an intention to kill yourself?" When the young person disclosed that he had already taken paracetamol, the final incremental question was for the psychiatrist to check if that disclosure constituted a suicide attempt by asking "have you ever done that", to which the young person confirmed that he had.

The important message therefore is that the final disclosure from the young person was not self-initiated. This shows how vital it is for practitioners to be prepared to ask these questions quite directly. However, to be able to ask a sensitive question directly and in a closed format, the incremental lead up is helpful to allow for this to happen. To summarise, there are useful practical ways you can ask a series of incremental questions to lead into discussions about risk with children and young people, for example:

- Start with general questions about feelings.
- Ask about coping strategies to manage those feelings.
- Clarify whether those coping strategies hurt the child or young person or anyone else.
- If the coping strategy hurts the child or young person ask further questions about recency, frequency, and severity.

- Ask about intentionality, that is, whether the purpose of the self-harm behaviour has been for emotional regulation or included suicidal intent (although it could be the case that the young person was ambivalent).
- Ask specifically about whether a behaviour with suicidal intent has already been engaged in.
- Pursue detail.

Normalising by externalising questions

Asking about self-harm or suicide using externalising questions projects it as merely a procedural standard requirement of the organisation. In doing so it normalises the topic as not specific to that child or young person but as relevant to all children and young people. Typically, an externalising question will be prefaced by an explicit statement that the question is one of a routine set of questions asked in this setting. In other words, this sets the question up as part of the organisational agenda, and not as a concern of the individual practitioner asking it. An advantage of this kind of question design is that it is a useful way of introducing a risk assessment question when there are no indicators of self-harm concern in the referral or in anything that the child or young person has said. This can also be especially helpful for practitioners whose primary professional role or training background does not include counselling/therapy skills.

To illustrate what externalising questions look like, we provide a data example from our paper (O'Reilly et al., 2016, p. 484). In this example a Community Psychiatric Nurse [CPN] is addressing a young person aged 17 years (taken from family 21 in the data).

Extract 2:

```
1. Prac → This is a question we have to ask everybody an'
2.          I'm sure that you've been asked it before (1.38)
3.          when you feel (0.92) a bit frustrated or a bit sad (0.63)
4.       → an' I know that you've punched walls before have you
5.          ever thought about (0.41) really hurting yourself
6. YP     No
```

There are different ways in which an externalising question can be formulated. In our example illustrated here, the practitioner had available some further information about the young person punching walls and this was used to move from the general to the specific. The key characteristic of this kind of question format is "we", "have to", and "everybody". These are important components of the question. The function of using the pronoun "we" is that it invokes the general non-personal organisation, where the practitioner is part of a wider collective rather than an individual seeking information. The use of "have to" removes the personal agency and introduces the question as a directive that is to be complied with. By stating that there is an imperative to ask "everybody" points to the idea that this young person is not being singled out. In other words, it frames the question as an inclusive question, merely as part of the assessment. This impersonal style is thus a useful technique for asking delicate or sensitive questions as it distances the asker from the question. In such a way, this distancing avoids disrupting alignment between the practitioner and young person by separating this tricky institutional question from other aspects of the social interaction. In this extract of data, the practitioner added some detail between the initial externalising component of the question and the self-harm (risk) part of the question:

- `I'm sure you've been asked it before (line 2)`
- `When you feel a bit frustrated or a bit sad (line 3)`
- `I know you've punched walls before (line 4)`

In this case, the practitioner did some further work to connect the general externalising question with the specific young person they are engaging. At first, the practitioner implied the normality of the question by suggesting the young person might have been asked it before ("I'm sure you've been asked this before"). What this suggests is that such a question is quite common. The second move was to suggest there may be occasions where emotions (frustrated/sad) result in certain behaviours (punching walls). By setting up this connection between emotion and behaviour provides a basis to ask about "hurting yourself".

To summarise, therefore, there are useful practical ways you can ask externalising or normalising questions to lead into discussions about risk with children and young people, for example:

- Externalise by using inclusive language such as "we" rather than the personal pronoun I.
- Externalise by stating that the question has to be asked; that there is an organisational expectation.
- Normalise by stating that everyone gets asked the question.
- Normalise by suggesting that the person may already have been asked a question like this before.

Both externalisation and normalisation strategies serve to present the asking the risk questions as standard procedure. Another way of enhancing the procedural and organisational directives of asking these questions might be to create a short-risk proforma. This visually represents the procedural nature of the institutional task.

Discussion

Through our analysis of child mental health assessments, we have identified two ways in which practitioners can ask risk questions. First, we have illustrated that one helpful way to ask about risk to self is to do so in an incremental manner, building from questions about emotions and behaviours toward more specific clarification about actual self-harm behaviour or suicidal ideation. Second, we have shown that an alternative approach is to ask a question in a way that removes agency and personalisation by externalising and normalising that question as a necessary procedural requirement of the organisation. There is no indication in the data to show that one was more effective than the other, rather they seemed to be used in different circumstances. That is, incremental questions tended to be used where the practitioner may have identified indications from the referral or the child or young person's comments that they may be at risk of self-harm. Externalising questions on the other hand, seemed to be used more often where there was no obvious indication for this kind of behaviour. In Box 6.1 we provide a practical summary of these communication strategies.

We have demonstrated the importance of asking children and young people about self-harm and their possible suicidal intentions as this is crucial in working toward the prevention of suicide in this population. However, asking children and young people risk-based questions in this area can

---

Box 6.1   Practical tips for communication

Practical tips for improving communication

- Bear in mind that a child or young person engaging in self-harm or suicidal ideation may not feel able to initiate a conversation about it (even in a help-seeking environment).
- The onus is on the practitioner to take responsibility for starting a dialogue.
- One way to ask about risk of harm to self is to steer the conversation in that direction incrementally.
- Alternatively, risk of harm to self can be talked about directly by prefacing the question with a caveat that the question is a procedural requirement of the organisation.
- If you have limited experience of asking these kinds of questions, it can be helpful to seek out support from your colleagues, supervisor, or manager.
- It is helpful to remember that the evidence shows that talking about self-harm and suicide does not worsen the situation, conversely it is shown to help.

be challenging, even in mental health settings where it is a necessary requirement of practice. Indeed, the quality of communication in healthcare is recognised to be one of the most important aspects of care and this is especially pertinent when working with children and young people (Stafford et al., 2016). Arguably, personal development of skills in communicating effectively around the important issues of risk is a professional and ethical priority (National Institute of Clinical Excellence, 2011). In this chapter, we have sought to bridge the gap between identified need from the literature and practice in the real world.

Implications and applications

A significant implication raised in this chapter is that in cases where children and young people are engaging in self-harm or have suicidal thoughts but choose not to disclose that, if they are never asked the question or the concern is never raised, they will go unsupported. Ultimately, this means that the behaviour and emotions are likely to escalate and could potentially have life-threatening consequences. Therefore, in situations where disclosure is not forthcoming, the onus is on the practitioner to introduce the topic. This is particularly true in the context of mental health assessments whereby risk assessments are a routine element of the process.

Arguably, it is important for practitioners to develop their skills and competencies in *how* to ask and *what* to say in asking those types of questions and through our analysis we have offered some practice-based suggestions. As practitioners build their skills and confidence in undertaking this task, hopefully there will be more opportunities for children and young people to talk about how they are feeling. The implications of this could be that talking about self-harm and suicide becomes a less taboo and stigmatised topic of conversation and becomes easier for practitioners to broach.

The use of recordings of conversations in real-world CAMHS settings has allowed us to shine a spotlight on what goes on in everyday mental health assessments and to work with the practitioners involved. Using this kind of naturally occurring data also provides opportunities for practitioners to reflect on theirs and their colleagues' practices to develop their skills and competencies in communication. Reflective practice is common in many professions and recording professional activities provides a forum for discussion, reflection, and personal development. If this is coupled with academic expertise, then further enhancement to the learning becomes possible on both sides. Such collaborative partnerships between practitioners and researchers can facilitate development of skills in all groups (O'Reilly and Parker, 2014). This collaborative approach is consistent with our methodological framework of Reflective Interventionist Conversation Analysis (O'Reilly et al., 2020).

Concluding remarks

Communication is a central guiding practice for most practitioners working with children and young people. By integrating clinical experience, academic knowledge, and language-based evidence we have provided an overview of an essential area of child and adolescent mental health, that of self-harm and suicide. To summarise, we have illustrated that the ways in which questions about self-harm and suicide are formulated can impact on the efficacy of the question in terms of eliciting responses. Both the incremental and externalising question design were found to successfully engage young people in these risk assessments. Although the data that this chapter was based on was from mental health services, the lessons learned from it are just as applicable to practitioners working in other settings, such as primary care and education. We suggest that teachers, social workers, general practitioners and so forth may find themselves in situations where they talk to children and young people about risk and an understanding of how to ask these questions sensitively could be useful. To help practitioners to have the skills and confidence to do so, communication about risk could be embedded in vocational training, or in further continuing professional development courses.

Clinical reflection: Dr Nikki Kiyimba (clinical psychologist)

As global statistics demonstrate, the prevalence of self-harm and suicide amongst children and young people (CYP) is of great concern for us all. Despite governments and non-profit organisations working hard to develop initiatives to reduce these statistics across the globe, the challenge remains very high and suicide rates are not decreasing as much as they should, and in some cases are increasing. It is well known that adverse childhood experiences (ACEs) including trauma and bullying are high on the list of contributing factors to increasing CYP vulnerability, and it is vital that we are all working hard to address these underlying issues that permeate through society whatever our professional role or context is.

In New Zealand, the 2019–2029 "Every Life Matters" action plan to reduce suicide is indicative of government commitment to tackling the problem at a societal level. For professionals on the "front line" working with individuals, families and whānau, reliable research is needed that provides concrete and applicable findings to support our day-to-day interactions with children and young people. It is a privilege for me to have the opportunity to span the space between clinical work as a psychologist, and academic work as a researcher and educator. It is this bridge that I feel passionate about, as we seek to make research accessible to all, so that we can learn how to be more effective in our professional practice. This chapter is a great example of the value of using live video recordings of mental health assessments to understand exactly how the difficult topics of self-harm and suicide risk are raised and discussed. One of the surprising findings was that in just over half of the assessments we analysed, professionals did *not* ask about risk. This therefore seems an obvious place to start our work to reduce suicide in young people – to ask.

There are different reasons why professionals do not ask these questions, one is a perception that the problem is not as huge as it really is, or that the problem does not exist here in my context where I work. The other is that there is a fear that bringing up the subject of self-harm or suicide with children and young people will give them ideas, and potentially encourage them to engage in risky behaviours. Both are false assumptions, and it is my hope that this chapter will help dispel these myths. Once we know that asking the questions is a vital piece in the jigsaw of reducing risk-taking behaviours, the next question is "How do we talk about risk?" What we have discussed are two styles of question design that have both been shown to be effective in encouraging children and young people to talk about risk with the professional asking the question. What we have learned is the importance of *what* we ask, and *how* we ask.

We are aware that children and young people are vulnerable to risk of harm from others, and indeed this may be one of the factors causing them to feel so distressed that they need to engage in life threatening behaviours. The research presented here just focuses on engaging in harm to self, and the findings provide us with tangible ways to just ask about risk in our next conversation with a child or young person.

Applying the incremental approach: In the data presented, one way to ask about risk of harm to self is incrementally; by starting with a question about emotions first, then to ask about behaviours that might be connected to or expressive of that emotion, and finally if self-harm is mentioned, to ask more about how and when etc. Where self-harm is present, a question about thoughts of suicide/ending your life can then be introduced. This approach has the advantage of engaging them in a conversation about their feelings and behaviours before talking about suicidal intent. It also allows the child or young person to navigate a difficult conversation in a structured way that is facilitated and scaffolded by the professional. Perhaps it is also a little easier for the professional to 'build up' to the suicide question in a way that feels more collaborative.

Applying the normalising and externalising approach: The second approach to asking about risk to self that was found to be effective in this data, was to say that there was a requirement of some sort on the professional to routinely ask all clients these questions about self-harm and suicide risk. This approach has the advantage that the topic can be raised very directly, which may be of value if the child or young person is difficult to engage in a more subtle incremental approach. It may also be useful in situations where time is limited and/or it is important to ensure the information is collected and recorded so appropriate support can be provided. Making the question embedded as a standard procedural practice also serves to normalise self-harm and suicide risk (unfortunately!), so they know that it is a topic that is OK to talk about with this person in this setting.

My view is that for most professionals who work with children and young people, it would be possible to use one or other of these types of question formats to introduce the topics of self-harm and suicide risk. Obviously, there is a need to be clear about the safeguarding protocols of the organisation within which we operate, and to be clear about what services or individuals we can refer them onto if a positive response to these questions is provided. This places the onus back on us to ensure we are aware of what these pathways are, so that we can be a small but extremely important part of the journey of that child or young person to finding healing and hope for their future.

References

American Psychiatric Association, 2013. *Diagnostic and Statistical Manual of Mental Disorders (Fifth ed) – DSM-5*. Washington, DC: American Psychiatric Association.

Appleby, L., Turnbull, P., Kapur, N., Gunnell, D., Hawton, K., 2019. New standard of proof for suicide at inquests in England and Wales. *BMJ 366* (8210), l4745.

Aseltine, R., James, A., Schilling, E., Glanovsky, J., 2007. Evaluating the SOS suicide prevention program: A replication and extension. *BMC Public Health 7*, 161.

Bajaj, P., Borreani, E., Ghosh, P., Methuen, C., Patel, M., Crawford, M., 2008. Screening for suicidal thoughts in primary care: The views of patients and general practitioners. *Ment. Health Family Med. 5*, 229–235.

Barrocas, A., Hankin, B., Young, J., Abela, J., 2012. Rates of nonsuicidal self-injury in youth: Age, sex, and behavioral methods in a community sample. *Pediatrics 130*, 39–45.

Björkenstam, E., Kosidou, K., Björkenstam, C., 2016. Childhood household dysfunction and risk of self-harm: A cohort study of 107 518 young adults in Stockholm County. *Int. J. Epidemiol. 45* (2), 501–511.

Bostik, K., Everall, R., 2006. In my mind I was alone: Suicidal adolescents' perceptions of attachment relationships. *Int. J. Adv. Counsell. 28*(3), 269–287.

Centres for disease Control and Prevention, 2019. Fatal Injury Reports, National, Regional and State, 1981–2017. https://webappa.cdc.gov/sasweb/ncipc/mortrate.html (accessed 11.09.2019).

Devon N. (2018a) We need to stop blaming social media for the teenage mental health crisis. https://metro.co.uk/2018/08/06/we-need-to-stop-blaming-social-media-for-the-teenage-mental-health-crisis7803618/amp/?ito=article.desktop.share.bottom.twitter&__twitter_impression=true.

Dazzi, T., Gribble, R., Wessely, S., Fear, N., 2014. Does asking about suicide and related behaviours induce suicide ideation? What is the evidence? *Psychological Med. 44*, 3361–3363.

Griffin, E., McMahon, E., McNicholas, F., Corcoran, P., Perry, I., Arensman, E., 2018. Increasing rates of self-harm among children, adolescents and young adults: A 10-year national registry study 2007–2016. *Soc. Psychiatry Psychiatr. Epidemiol. 53* (7), 663–671.

Hawton, K., Saunders, K., O'Connor, R., 2012. Self-harm and suicide in adolescents. *Lancet 379*, 2373–2382.

Kiyimba, N., Lester, J., O'Reilly, M., 2019. *Using naturally occurring data in health research: A practical guide.* Springer.

Kiyimba, N., O'Reilly, M., 2018. Reflecting on what "you said" as a way of reintroducing difficult topics in child mental health assessments. *Child. Adolesc. Ment. Health 23* (3), 148–154.

Mars, B., Klonsky, E., Moran, P., O'Connor, R., Tilling, K., Wilkinson, P., Gunnell, D., 2019. Predictors of future suicide attempt among adolescents with suicidal thoughts or non-suicidal self-harm: A population-based birth cohort study. *Lancet Psychiatry 6*, 327–337.

Marshall, P., 2015. Seven-year olds treated for self-harming as number of cases among primary school children rises 10%. https://www.itv.com/news/2015-10-13/seven-year-olds-treated-for-self-harming-as-number-of-cases-among-primary-school-children-rises-10/ (accessed 09.11.2020).

Mash, E., Hunsley, 2005. Special section: Developing guidelines for the evidence-based assessment of child and adolescent disorders. *J. Child. Adolesc. Psychol. 34* (3), 362–379.

Ministry of Health, 2019. Suicide facts: 2016 data (provisional). Wellington: Ministry of Health. www.health.govt.nz/publication/suicide-facts-2016-data-provisional (accessed 16.10.2019).

National Institute of Clinical Excellence, 2004. *The Short-Term Physical and Psychological Management and Secondary Prevention of Self-Harm in Primary and Secondary Care.* NICE, London.

National Institute of Clinical Excellence, 2011. *Self-Harm in Over 8s: Short-Term Management and Prevention of Recurrence NICE guidelines [CG133].* NICE, London.

National Institute of Mental Health, 2020. Suicide. https://www.nimh.nih.gov/health/statistics/suicide.shtml (accessed 12.10.2020).

NHS Digital, 2018. Mental health of children and young people in England, 2017: Summary of key findings. https://files.digital.nhs.uk/F6/A5706C/MHCYP%202017%20Summary.pdf (accessed 11.12.2018).

Office for National Statistics, 2016. Deaths registered in England and Wales (Series DR). https://www.one.gov.uk/peoplepopulationandcommunity/birthsdeathsandmarriages/deaths/bulletins/deathsregisteredinenglandandwalesseriesdr/2016). (accessed 22.09.2019).

O'Reilly, M., Kiyimba, N., Karim, K., 2016. 'This is a question we have to ask everyone': Asking young people about self-harm and suicide. *J. Psychiatr. Ment. Health Nurs. 23*, 479–488.

O'Reilly, M., Kiyimba, N., Lester, J., Muskett, T., 2020. Reflective Interventionist Conversation Analysis. *Discourse & Communication 14* (6), 619–634.

O'Reilly, M., Parker, N., 2014. *Doing Mental Health Research with Children and Adolescents: A Guide to Qualitative Methods.* SAGE, London.

Reeves, A., 2010. *Counselling Suicidal Clients.* SAGE, London.

Simms, C., Scowcroft, E., 2018. *Suicide Statistics Report: Latest Statistics for the UK and Republic of Ireland.* Samaritans, London.

Stafford, V., Hutchby, I., Karim, K., O'Reilly, M., 2016. "Why are you here?" Seeking children's accounts of their presentation to CAMHS. *Clin. Child. Psychol. Psychiatry 21* (1), 3–18.

Swannell, S., Martin, G., Page, A., et al., 2014. Prevalence of nonsuicidal self-injury in nonclinical samples: Systematic review, meta-analyses and meta-regression. *Suicide Life Threat. Behav. 44*, 273–303.

World Health Organization, 2010. Intervention guide for mental, neurological and substance use disorders in non-specialized health settings: Version 1.0. Geneva: World Health Organization. http://whqlibdoc.who.int/publications/2010/9789241548069_eng.pdf (accessed 23.04.2014).

World Health Organization, 2014. *Preventing Suicide: A Global Imperative.* WHO, Luxembourg.

World Health Organization, 2016. International classification of diseases. as retrieved from https://icd.who.int/browse10/2016/en#/X60-X84 (accessed 09.11.2020).

World Health Organization, 2019. *Suicide in the World: Global Health Estimates.* WHO, Geneva.

Zetterqvist, M., 2015. The DSM-5 diagnosis of nonsuicidal self-injury disorder: a review of the empirical literature. *Child Adolesc. Psychiatry Ment. Health 9*, 31–44.

Chapter 7

Communicating with parents about psychotropic medication treatment

F. Alethea Marti and Bonnie T. Zima

Introduction

The core of child psychiatry is the therapeutic relationship between the provider and the family. Mental health practitioners seek to develop treatment plans that will improve the child's quality of life and lead to better long-term outcomes, and it is highly rewarding to see one's patients achieve long-term success in school, in friendships, and in family relationships, months or even years later.

Parents and primary caregivers play a key role in treatment success: because they see the child every day, they are able to monitor symptoms and track behavioural problems, as well as make in-the-moment decisions about managing these problems. For this reason, treatment success requires a strong relationship of mutual trust and shared goals between parent[1] and provider (Brinkman and Epstein, 2011). If parents do not trust providers, treatment adherence will be low and the likelihood of drop-out will increase. Similarly, if providers feel they cannot rely upon parents for accurate observations about the child, they will not have the necessary information to diagnose or monitor treatment effectiveness. For this reason, it is crucial that providers work to build mutual trust and a relationship that is non-judgmental and allows parents to express their fears and concerns, so that both parties can work together to develop best treatment options tailored for the family.

In this chapter, we focus specifically on the relationship between parent and psychiatrist during psychotropic medication titration, the process by which a new medication is gradually administered in order to determine the ideal dose needed by the child. While these strategies can be used more generally, it is important to note the ways in which medication titration differs from other forms of mental health treatment (such as therapy):

1   Providers can face resistance from parents to the idea of a long-term prescription medication, including concerns about side-effects, addiction, or having it become a gateway to illegal drug use later in life. For psychotropic medications, there are additional fears of personality

changes or distrust at "fixing" a behavioural problem with chemicals. In our interviews with families for this study, a common theme that emerged was parents' concerns that the medication would suppress the child's natural enthusiasm or reduce them to a listless "zombie" state (see also Bussing et al., 2012; Hansen and Hansen, 2006; Travell and Visser, 2006).

2   Most of the treatment process occurs outside the psychiatrist's office. The parent bears the primary burdens of administering daily medication, closely monitoring the child for bad reactions, and making immediate decisions if these occur. While some parents may prefer to have the child's welfare in their own hands rather than that of a stranger, others may feel they are being given a medical role for which they are untrained.

Despite these differences, we anticipate that the strategies and tips we present here are also useful for other types of child treatment, particularly cases where there is strong fear or stigma, or where a caregiver is required to implement treatments between clinic visits or track the child's condition on a daily basis.

The significance of parent/provider communication: Context and literature review

Across multiple care settings, family perception of good communication and rapport with the child's provider are connected with other positive outcomes such as greater engagement in treatment, increased therapeutic alliance, better adherence to medication and treatment, higher parental satisfaction, and increased comfort discussing psychosocial concerns, all of which lead to better mental health care outcomes (Schoenthaler et al., 2009; Hart et al., 2007; Nobile and Drotar, 2003; Tarn et al., 2006; Wissow et al., 2010). For minority and immigrant families, good "cultural congruence" (shared cultural understandings between provider, patient or parent, and interpreter if there is one) is also key to successful communication, and can increase the likelihood of positive treatment outcomes for Latinos and Hispanics regardless of language fluency (Costantino et al., 2009; Villalobos et al., 2016).

In contrast, when parent feel that communication with their provider is poor, there is an increased likelihood of treatment drop-out, low medication adherence, misinformation, or mental illness stigma (Arcia et al., 2004; Bussing et al., 2007; Yeh et al., 2005; Zima et al., 2010). This effect becomes exacerbated for parents from racial or ethnic minority backgrounds (Arcia et al., 2004; Bussing et al., 2007), where differing paradigms of illness, caregiving, or even normal child behaviour may cause conflicts between family and provider (Ojeda et al., 2011) and lead to reluctance to seek out institutional care, especially if parents feel social stigma from medical authorities (Yeh et al., 2005).

Good communication is not always achieved, however. In an examination of US acute care visits, only one-third (32%) of providers even attempted to elicit other concerns patients might have apart from their initial complaint. Those providers who did so were more likely to receive a response if asking early in the appointment rather than at the end (Robinson et al., 2016). In medication titration visits, eliciting other concerns is important for two reasons. First, seemingly unrelated physical or behavioural problems may actually be side effects (e.g., insomnia) or indicators of medication ineffectiveness. Second, medication treatment is only part of the provider's larger goal to improve the child's quality of life. In addition to focusing on medication, the providers in our study would often also advise parents on other problems, such as creating effective homework or bedtime routines.

Importance of good communication in medication treatment

Positive medication outcomes over time depend on two factors: continuing to use the prescribed medication regularly (medication adherence) and continuing to meet with a provider to monitor changes or problems and receive refills (clinic attendance). Both factors are almost entirely in the hands of primary caregivers.

The degree to which patients and family are open to or resistant toward medication treatments varies cross-culturally even within a shared language. For example, Stivers and colleagues found that UK patients are more resistant to prescription medication, while US patients are more likely to expect prescriptions (Stivers and Barnes, 2017), and that providers frame recommendations accordingly, with UK providers using more inclusive language (offers or proposals, rather than authoritative pronouncements) to elicit patients' agreement (Stivers et al., 2018).

Supporting medication recommendations: Research findings

In this chapter, we examine strategies that child psychiatrists use to encourage parent engagement and buy-in toward medication recommendations, and illustrate how parents, psychiatrists, and sometimes children, discuss and make decisions about necessary changes in medication such as increasing a dose or switching to a new prescription. We particularly highlight ways doctors strategically set up their recommendations to give parents active power in the decision-making process and provide a non-judgmental space to express fears and concerns.

The transcripts presented in this chapter are from video-recordings of child psychiatry appointments for children diagnosed with attention deficit/hyperactivity disorder (ADHD) starting on first-time stimulant medication (see inset). We examined the first three follow-up appointments after initial diagnosis as this is the crucial early stage when groundwork for the psychiatrist/parent/child relationship is developed and when parents' and children's concerns about medication are most apparent. Data were collected for a feasibility study of an ADHD medication titration web app designed to help improve communication between parents and providers about children's symptoms and side effects (Mikesell et al., 2018; see Box 7.1).

Presenting the medication recommendation

In these appointments, providers are negotiating three main goals:

1 To provide quality evidence-based care for the child;
2 To engage the parent as an active participant in the decision-making process; and
3 To allow parents room to express fears or concerns and acknowledge these in a non-judgmental fashion.

In some cases, these goals may appear to be in conflict. For example, if a parent's fears about medication are based on misinformation, the provider

---

Box 7.1 Web App Feasibility Study

- **Site:** Two child psychiatry clinics in Los Angeles, California, USA, serving low-income, primarily minority families

- **Research Participants:**

  o 21 English-speaking parents of children aged 5–11 years
  o Child is diagnosed with ADHD and prescribed stimulant medication for the first time

- **Data Collected:**

  o Video recordings of the first 3 appointments after receiving the prescription
  o After-visit questionnaires about medication acceptability, parental confidence, and satisfaction with treatment
  o Open-ended interviews with parents and providers, and ethnographic observations of clinic workflow

- **Goals:** To test the feasibility and acceptability of a web app designed to track parent/teacher reports of symptoms and side effects and to assist parents and providers in discussing them during medication titration visits

- **See also:** Mikesell et al. (2018)

will typically focus on building rapport and addressing the parent's concerns (goal #3) before correcting their misinformation (goal #1). We therefore provide some practical tips in Box 7.2.

Four types of support for a medication decision

When presenting a medication recommendation, doctors frequently offered some form of support for their decision. In our research, these fell into four categories:

*   **Observations of symptoms and side effects,** based on parents' or teachers' reports. (Less frequently, doctors may cite their own observations of a child's behaviour during the appointment.)
*   **Parent or child's preferences or dislikes,** for example a parent not wanting a high dose or a child not liking how the medication makes them feel.
*   **Hypothetical future scenarios** in which doctors describe different possible ways a dose change might play out (e.g., "if we see improvement, then ... otherwise ...")
*   **Expert medical knowledge** about ADHD or stimulant medication.

Each type of support can be used strategically to include parents as partners in the treatment process, making them active collaborators in decision-making and creating a non-judgmental environment where their concerns and fears can be addressed.

Medication recommendations supported by parent observations

Excerpt 1: First follow-up visit.

1. DOC: The other thing is, <u>since she's been more irritable on the weekends</u>, I would just keep the Concerta [medication] going. On the weekends.

Because ADHD symptoms occur in a variety of contexts, providers heavily depend on the observations of adults who spend lengthy periods of time with the child, such as parents and teachers. When making recommendations about dose changes, providers often reference parents' own reports (e.g., more irritable on the weekends). Building on information presented by the parent adds strength to the provider's recommendation. Such repetition also emphasizes the key role the parent plays in the treatment process as the person in charge of monitoring the child's status.

Box 7.2   Practical tips

Practical tips for improving communication during treatment recommendation

- Throughout the entire process, create opportunities for shared treatment decision-making with the parent.
- When giving your recommendation, explicitly show that it is consistent with the parent or child's preferences and concerns, or that it is based on information they provided (e.g., reports of symptoms).
- Depending on cultural and class factors, parents may feel uncomfortable contradicting an authority figure even if they disagree with you. Frame the interaction as an equal partnership by using:

  o   inclusive *we* and *you*-focused language (*we can decrease the dose* rather than *I can prescribe a lower dose*).
  o   mitigating phrases (*I think; maybe we can; let's try*), rather than authoritative ones (*you need to*).
  o   check-in questions to see how parent and child feel about each step (*how does that sound? are you okay with that?*)

- If parents are uncomfortable with a best practice treatment recommendation:

  o   Don't dismiss their fears as "wrong" or unrealistic. Instead, emphasize your shared priorities as a team (see above) and work together to address their concerns (see below).
  o   Focus on the source of the parent's discomfort: can you plan in advance or safely change the recommendation to alleviate it? (e.g., if the parent is worried about accidental overmedicating, suggest a very gradual titration).
  o   Offer clear strategies for addressing different future scenarios (e.g., "we'll go back to the lower dose if the stomachaches don't go away after three days"), especially for scenarios that the parent is worried about.
  o   Empower the parent in this process: remind them that they know their child best, that you're relying on them to make the in-the-moment decisions if any problems emerge (e.g., whether to skip a dose when the child is ill), and how they can contact you if they have questions.

Excerpt 2: Mother and son's second follow-up visit. Mother has just finished describing problems the child is having with distractibility during homework time.

1. DOC: I see, okay. So sounds like, um, um, maybe we could do better medwise –
2. MOM: Mhm.
3. DOC: – as far as, um, you know, helping with focus and attention, and – helping him to be less distracted.
4. MOM: Mhm.
5. DOC: Um, I wonder if. You know we could try a higher dose
6. the reason we didn't do it last time is cuz
7. we were concerned about side effects
8. he was having those headaches and stuff?
9. MOM: Mhm
10. DOC: But now that he's not having them. You know, I think –
11. It sounds like – you know we COULD go that way.

Rather than repeating the parent's observations as in Excerpt 1, this doctor begins with the referential phrase *sounds like*, to tie her upcoming recommendation to the information the parent has just given her. She also strategically uses language that encourages Mom to become an active decision-maker. Repeatedly using *we* rather than *I* frames her recommendation as a joint decision (*we could, we were concerned*). She also downplays her position of authority by using hedge words – mitigating modifiers that make one's speech sound less assertive and more hesitant: *I wonder if, it sounds like, we could.*

Medication recommendations supported by parent/child preferences

Excerpt 3: Third follow-up visit with Anna.[2] Doctor is recommending an increased medication dose, but Mother is reluctant.

1. DOC: But it – you know, um, but you're seeing benefits ((nodding)) from the medication.
2. MOM: ((nods)) Yes.
3. DOC: But you're afraid to go up too high cuz you don't want it [her personality] to completely change, yeah.
4. MOM: Yeah.
5. KID: Change what?
6. DOC: And we, we don't want that either. We want her to still be engaged and –
7. MOM: And happy.

Parent and child preferences were given equal weight to observable symptoms and side effects as reasons to change or maintain a dose. By explicitly referring to a parent (or child's) worries, the doctor turns her professional recommendation into a collaborative decision where the parent's input has equal value. This strategy can be effective in defusing disagreements if parents' preferences contradict medical best practice, and can open the door to conversations about how to adjust medication recommendations to address parents' concerns.

In this example, rather than contradicting Mom's factual understanding of how titration works, the doctor first addresses the underlying reason for her reluctance and reassures her that they both share the same priority: neither of them wants to alter the child's personality, they want her to stay her happy, engaged self. By emphasizing these shared goals, the doctor tries to allay the parent's resistance to her recommendation. Near the end of same visit, the doctor returns to the topic and says she would like to "try a higher dose" (see excerpt 6) and the parent eventually agrees.

Eliciting children's preferences

Younger children in our study were not heavily involved in medication decision-making; indeed, doctors sometimes had trouble getting clear responses from a young child about "how the med feels" or "what it's helping you with". However, older children did understand and could participate in the conversation by describing side effects or school successes or by stating their own concerns. (See Travell and Visser, 2006, for more about the importance of including the perspectives of youth in ADHD medication treatment.)

The following two excerpts follow Keith, who has just begun a medication that is effective in controlling his symptoms but also causes problematic headaches. We see how psychiatrist and mother both use inclusive language to validate Keith as a participant in the decision-making process.

Excerpt 4: First follow-up. Mother relays Keith's preferences to Doctor.

1. MOM: When I ask him, you know, "Okay if the medication's making you feel this way, do you want to continue to take it?"
2. I'm like "Mommy's not gonna force you to take it".
3. DOC: Mhm?
4. MOM: And he was like "No, I'll stay on it". And I said "Okay".
5. Cuz I've asked him on numerous occasions, y'know, how he's feeling?
6. DOC: Yeah?
7. MOM: Um, y'know "Do you want to continue with the medication?"

8. DOC: Yeah.
9. MOM: He says he don't wanna stop.
10. DOC: Okay. *((to KID))* You – you like what it's doing for you then?
11. KID: *((nods))*
12. DOC: Overall you like it. Okay. Well we're gonna help you try to see if we can deal with some of the – some of the side effects, okay?

In a situation with the potential for a very imbalanced power dynamic (one child speaking to two adults) mother and doctor both work to make sure Keith's perspective is included and respected. Keith is a quiet child who says very little during appointments. Here, his mother voices his concerns and preferences by relaying conversations she had with him in private. Afterwards, the doctor addresses Keith directly to confirm their accuracy (lines 10–12).

Excerpt 5: Second follow-up. Doctor discusses with Mom the possibility of a higher dose now that Keith's headaches have decreased.

10 DOC *((to Kid))*: What do you – I know you mentioned that that's was something you'd be okay with, what do you think, Keith?
11 KID *((looks up))*: Um.
12 *((pause while DOC looks at KID))*
13 KID: Uhhh, yeah?
14 DOC: Would you be – Um. I was wondering if you'd be okay with maybe, trying a higher dose of the medicine? To see if it might help you focus more.
15 KID: *((nods slightly))* Yeah.
16 DOC: Would that be something you'd be open to trying?
17 KID: *((nods a bit more vigorously))*
18 DOC: Cuz, we could try it and then you could let us know what you think.
19 KID: *((nods))*
20 DOC: Okay?
21 KID: *((nods again, smiling))*

Similar to Excerpt 2, the doctor uses inclusive *we-* and *you*-focused language, check-in questions, and mitigating hedges (*we could, would you be okay with*) to include Mom and Keith in both the decision-making and the treatment implementation. Additionally, by repeatedly using the verb "to try" (lines 14–16), she presents the medication change as a temporary experiment that can be stopped at any time, not as a weighty final decision. Keith appears to not be paying attention at first, but soon agrees with nods and smiles (lines 17–21).

Medication recommendations supported by hypothetical futures

In contrast to behavioural observations or preferences, a third strategy used by the child psychiatrists is to describe alternative scenarios that could result from a dose increase. These hypotheticals are often presented as pairs of if/then/else statements, contrasting good and bad futures, as we can see in the following conversation, which revisits the family from Excerpt 3:

Excerpt 6: Third follow-up. Anna is responding well to the medication.

1. DOC: Well, the reason I wanna try it is just to see.
2. So we would try the 27 [mg dose]
3. and if you say - if teacher says "Wow she's doing so much better even -"
4. MOM: ((nodding))
5. DOC: And there's not any side effects
6. then we say "Okay maybe we should try this dose".
7. Cuz, um, if you're saying "Noo there's not an improvement", and there's more side effects?
8. We would go back down. To the other one.
9. We would know in a couple days.
10. MOM: Mm.

In this excerpt, the doctor presents two possible futures, each with a medication plan:

- Future #1 (lines 3–5): Parent and teacher see improvement, no side effects.

    o   Medication plan (line 6): Continue with the higher dose.

- Future #2 (line 7): No improvement, more side effects.

    o   Medication plan (line 8): Go back to the lower dose.

By presenting both possibilities at the same time, the parent is not pressured to make a high-stakes decision about her child's well-being – both paths remain open to her even after the child starts on the higher dose.

Interestingly, the doctor's description of these two futures relies on data to be collected by the parent herself (either through direct observation or talking to the teacher), thereby placing Mom in charge of the experiment: she will talk to the teacher and see if the new dose is effective, she will monitor the child for side effects, and, if there are problems, she has the authority to say "Noo there's not an improvement" (line 7) and reverse the decision. With all these verbal framings, the doctor sets herself up as an advisor supporting the parent, rather than as the medical authority in charge. Mom retains responsibility and control over what's best for her child.

Medication recommendations based on medical knowledge

Excerpt 7: First follow-up. Parent and child have been describing child's improved school performance.

1. DOC: So you feel like you – how do you feel the medication helps?
2. KID: A little bit good.
3. DOC: A little bit good? What do you notice? You're the expert.

Medical expertise was the least frequent reason doctors used to support a recommended dose change. Even though they have superior knowledge about ADHD treatment and stimulant medication, they actively found way to diminish the potential imbalance in authority, positioning parents (and older children) as equal collaborators or sometimes even as the final decision-makers. When doctors did cite medical expertise, it was typically in an educational fashion, giving parents more information about ADHD or the medication so they can make better decisions.

Excerpt 8: First follow-up. Doctor and parent have been talking about child's school performance and relationship with siblings.

1. DOC: We can make this decision over time
2. But y'know some kids do end up needing a second dose as the day wears on.
3. Because you know their teachers are noticing in the afternoon they're not as focused, they're having hyperactivity.
4. So there's certainly room to make adjustments like that.
5. Um, are you noticing that by the time she's home she's more hyperrr is there anything?
6. MOM: Yes.
7. DOC: Okay.
8. MOM: I notice that by the time she's home, she's ((hand gesture)) – off. I noticed it because of the weekend.

Here the doctor presents background information about ADHD medication to help contextualize what the parent and child have noticed. However, she quickly turns the conversation back to the parent's own observations (line 5).

Guidance for evidence-based practice

To provide quality evidence-based care, providers must not only apply their own medical expertise about best practices, but also build parent trust and openness. As we emphasized earlier, good treatment outcomes depend on parents being actively on-board: they are the ones scheduling therapy or doctor's appointments, administering medications, monitoring the child, and other tasks such as therapy "homework".

Building such trust requires giving parents a non-judgmental setting where they can express concerns and fears without feeling like they are dumb or silly, even when such concerns seem irrelevant or medically inaccurate (e.g., believing that ADHD medication is a gateway to illegal drug use). In some cases, parent resistance may stem from outside sources: cultural or community norms, or the conflicting views of other family members. Building this safe space of trust will allow parents and providers to work together to address such sensitive issues (see also Smoliak et al., this volume).

The provider's goal is to secure parents' uptake, engagement in treatment, and sustaining treatment after the initial learning phase ends (e.g., continuing to give the medication after titration or to use the cognitive behaviour therapy (CBT) techniques after the training class ends). Here are five practices to assist in developing those goals:

1 Clarify your reasons for making a recommendation

Although it may seem redundant, reiterating what a parent has told you will make transparent the logic behind your decisions and emphasize the parent's role in the decision-making.

2 Explicitly cite the parent's input

"Referential phrases" indicate the source from which you learned a fact (for example: *the teacher said* or *what I'm hearing from you*). Whether you are citing a behavioural observation or a parent preference, using referential phrases to explicitly highlight the parent/child as the information source helps emphasise that your own recommendations are consistent with their experiences.

3 Use future hypotheticals to acknowledge different problems that may occur and how they will be handled

Doctors in our study used if-then-else scenarios to assure parents that there would be a plan in place for dealing with future problems. Quite often, the plan for the "negative" future was to revert to a previous dose. Emphasising this option ahead of time decreases the sense of risk parents may feel in trying a higher dose in the first place.

4 Engage the parent as an active collaborator in solving these future problems

Child ADHD treatment relies heavily on observations from parents and teachers who see the child's everyday life outside of the psychiatrist's office. When providers present hypothetical future scenarios (see above), they give parents the major role of on-the-ground observer, collecting the data on the child's status that will determine the final medication decision.

5 Also apply these strategies to include older children as decision-makers

Requesting the child's input helps them learn to be more aware of how the medication affects their mind and body. Encouraging them to ask questions can decrease fear of trying a new dose by reassuring the child that both doctor and parent will take their concerns seriously if anything goes wrong. (For example: one child worried that the medication would cause her to gain weight.)

In the next section, we examine the reasons and rewards in building professional relationships with families from the clinician's perspective.

Reflections of a child psychiatrist: Engaging with parents and children over time

The essence of practicing child psychiatry is the therapeutic relationship between the practitioner and both the child and the adults who are influential in his or her care over time. Like our colleagues in paediatrics, we aim to maintain relationships with the child and their family that last across developmental phases, that change as the child grows, and that may last through adolescence and into adulthood. Some of my patients continue to return to me well into college. They make appointments for when they are home during spring break or Thanksgiving, rather than seeking out a new adult psychiatrist, because this clinic is their home and we are part of the family. Watching these children excel and grow and celebrating their successes with them is one of the great rewards of my profession.

As child psychiatrists, we are often the "last stop" for parents with concerns about their child's mental health. Many parents who come to us are reluctant about long-term medication or worry the child may be labelled as "defective" if they are receiving psychiatric care. For this reason, it is crucial to start building trust from the beginning. If the first appointment doesn't go well, the parent may never return.

There is often a "tipping point" for parents that stimulates recognition of a problem that requires seeking care outside their usual support networks. It typically occurs around 9 years of age, because academic demands increase in fourth grade when application of basic reading and math skills begins. In the case of very young child with developmental delays or symptoms across the spectrum of autism, contact may be sooner. Tipping points can also occur later in life, for example the transitions to middle school, high school, preparing for standardized tests for college, or transition to college. For older children, the stronger relationship may be between psychiatrist and child rather than psychiatrist and parent.

The initial visit: Understanding concerns and gathering information

Because the initial visit is so important, it is paramount to begin the session with open-ended questions. We explore why the family is here, what concerns they have, and what treatment or services they seek. Depending on the age of the child, parent preferences, and the child's comfort level, we might gather information from multiple perspectives. Father, mother, other primary caregiver, and child or teen often have different but equally valuable perspectives of how need for care is conceptualised (or not) and the goals for care.

The provider's own goals are to understand parent and child concerns, gather information to support or rule-out diagnoses, and be open to observations that may not fit diagnostic criteria but nevertheless could indicate target symptoms or areas of functional impairment that will be useful to detect clinical improvement. An additional goal is to create an environment where both parent and child are free to express their worries without fear of judgement, as we discussed in this chapter.

Working together to "name" the problem

As we formulate the diagnosis together with the parent's input, there should be additional ongoing back and forth with the family to further clarify symptoms, their duration, frequency, and context. During this process, the we work to validate the child's or parent's concerns and to further revise, reframe, and test diagnoses. This is an opportunity to provide consultation to the parent and/or child about the "name" for the concern, or set of concerns, they have brought to the psychiatrist. This may lead to further discussion when parents or children ask additional questions and bring their fears to light about the implications of a diagnosis.

Often, a child will have multiple comorbid diagnoses, and so we must decide together with the family which one to address first. Sometimes it may be the one that most distresses the child. Another strategy is to start with the diagnosis that has the most wide-ranging effects – for example, often a child's anxiety symptoms will decrease once their ADHD symptoms are controlled. Sometimes there may be practical considerations, for example working with a family to treat ADHD symptoms while waiting for a confirmation of an autism diagnosis that would allow the mother to request additional services from the school. As trust increases, other topics of discussion will arise including cultural differences, intergenerational differences (e.g., parent versus grandparent views about the child), and sometimes parental misinformation, becoming an opportunity to provide guidance when it can align with the parent's or child's timing.

Working together to develop a treatment plan

With a diagnosis, we next develop a treatment plan that is guided by treatment guidelines or practice parameters. Usually we offer first-line treatment options to the parent, and then listen to their initial impressions. Parents' and children's receptivity to starting a medication prescription will vary. Often, they worry about the effects of chronic medication, or they do not want their child being labelled as "defective" by others. Once again, the relationship between the provider and family is paramount. It's a culmination of timing and readiness and trust. If the parent is indecisive, or if both parents disagree, I will offer other options and remind them that the clinic is here for them whenever they are ready. Interim options if parents are not ready for medication include: parent training, starting (or continuing) therapy, or school-based interventions like tutoring or coaching. We provide additional time for parents to do their own research, seek advice from others, or talk more at home as a family. We also provide further education about medication treatment such as expected effects, common side effects, and treatment logistics.

The overarching goal in such education is to prepare the parent and child for what to expect in a medication trial, and set the groundwork for open communication, especially if side effects persist or more serious ones emerge. Psychotropic medication is often effective but is dependent on parents' administering the medication regularly and over time. Opening discussions with parents reinforces the depth of the relationship, which also improves adherence to recommended care and the likelihood of effective treatment.

Developing the relationship over time

The relationship between parent, child and psychiatrist matures over multiple visits. We tailor the nuances of treatment decisions based on factors such as the child's sensitivity to side effects, a parent's desire for a slower titration of medication, or parent or child's comfort level with medication. We tend to see this comfort level increase as parents notice improvement such as less tension at home and school related to a child's reduction in hyperactivity, better school reports, or a child's symptoms of major depression improving.

As the parent and child's concerns are reassured over multiple follow-up visits, we can shift to building rapport over improvements. I make opportunities to praise the child for the efforts they have made and to personalize the milestones they have achieved, and encourage parents to do the same. "We're so proud of you. The teacher says you're raising your hand in class now". "It's great that you got chosen for the soccer team". Acknowledging successes creates a cyclical reinforcement of recommended care and clinical improvement that ideally is perpetuated over time.

During middle school and high-school, I frequently spend more time talking to the child rather than the parent. Sometimes, as children become more independent, they think they no longer need the medication, and the parent may be reluctant to force them to take it. I explain that I will start treating them like the older high-school and college kids. I will be asking for their own impressions now rather than depending on Mom's reports. I tell them, "Only you know how well you're concentrating or paying attention. Only you know which subjects are hard for you in school and whether the medication is working or if we need to try something else". An eighth or ninth grader wants to be treated like they're grown up. They want that respect. The provider/child relationship should change over time as the child matures.

Tending to the development and preservation of these relationships, both with the child and those influential in their life, is paramount amidst the delivery of the care processes required for psychotropic medication evaluation and follow-up. Tailoring the treatment to the clinical needs of the child and his or her family will improve the likelihood of effective care. There is also an invaluable sense of purpose and personal reward in establishing long-term relationships with the patients we care for, their families, and others who are influential in their development, and in watching these children achieve and excel over the years.

Why caring for children with psychiatric disorders and their families is so rewarding to me

I was attracted to the medical profession because I have always wanted to help others. What drew me away from internal medicine and into psychiatry was the type of relationship with the patient and the type of care I could provide. To me, the essence of a human is the mind and soul. Over the years, this pivotal moment has protected me from the "burn-out" that many physicians experience.

When I began in child psychiatry it seemed to me that the mental health of children was minimized and the early classification systems for psychiatric diagnoses applied more to adults. Early research in child psychiatry focused on validating ADHD as a disorder and proving that stimulant medication was effective in reducing target symptoms. Diagnostic criteria for major depression, bipolar disorder, and post-traumatic stress disorder included "more adult-like symptoms" that did not account for the development of children. However, over time, more research emerged and diagnostic criteria flexed to include symptoms such as chronic irritability as an indicator of depression in a child. There was increasing awareness that onset of mood disorders, anxiety disorders, and psychosis often occurred prior to adulthood. Conversely, adults suffering from chronic inattention, difficulties focusing and sustaining mental tasks to organize and complete their work, were validated as having ADHD and thus able to access stimulant medication treatment to reduce their suffering.

Likewise, when I started my career in child psychiatry it seemed that the impact of exposure to trauma was also minimised, although, of course, the seriousness of child neglect and physical and sexual abuse were recognised. However, over the years there has been more acceptance of the negative impact of verbal abuse, abrupt separation from parents, bullying, and putting children in social situations for which they are unprepared and unprotected.

Young boys especially are allowed more to have feelings of anxiety, depression, or simply not feel "ready" for a developmental step. Adolescent girls battling major depression, eating disorders, and urges to "cut" are now less likely to be dismissed. During my career, our profession is realising that yes there are psychiatric disorders in children, they start early, are treatable, and could even be prevented if we respond quickly to repair the emotional sequelae of even mild trauma exposure.

Another reward of this profession is meeting and working with so many amazing parents, grandparents, and other primary caregivers. Families come to us as a last stop and are often reluctant about the medication. They want the best for their child, but no parent wants their child to have a psychiatric condition or to be on chronic medication. On the other hand, we also have families where more than one child and a parent have ADHD, so when the second child manifests symptoms the mother is on it early. They know it's a family risk factor, they feel empowered to manage it, and they continue loving their children without a negative label.

The children go through so much as they grow and mature. One of my recent patients was very bright but struggling in 9th grade because of ADHD. She did not have hyperactivity, but she had the inattention. Now she's going to UC Berkeley, feeling confident and making plans to continue her ADHD care through student health services.

It is also a journey with each child. The child keeps changing with their development which is uniquely timed for each person. The parent's comfort level increases as well, and they will parent differently if it's a first, second, or third child. Marriages, jobs, and stresses on the family all change over time. The provider is part of this journey. In a very real sense, we become a small part of the family's journey. Their willingness to trust me with the care of their loved one, turn to me for guidance and support, and even challenge me to better understand, is rich, rewarding, and sustaining. I am grateful to have a career that allows me to have these types of relationships with my patients.

Conclusion

In order to achieve positive treatment outcomes and improved quality of life for the child, it is crucial to build a collaborative relationship of trust and rapport between provider and family. Because medical professionals are sometimes perceived as authority figures, providers may have to take active steps to reframe this relationship as a more equal one where parents feel comfortable expressing concerns and contributing to the decision-making, and where providers work to take those concerns into account when developing best practice treatment plans. This can be achieved by using inclusive language, backing medication decisions with input previously provided by parents, and reminding parents that they oversee monitoring the child's status and have authority to make in-the-moment decisions if anything unexpected happens. Similar strategies can be used to involve older children in describing how the medications feel and affect their own behaviour, as well as reassuring them that their concerns will be listened to.

Developing trust and openness between provider, parent, and child, not only improves medication outcomes, it also contributes to an ongoing relationship which will support children's long-term success in school and life.

Notes

1 For readability we use the term "parent" throughout this chapter; the families in our research study also included grandmothers, aunts, and one great-grandmother, who were primarily or solely responsible for raising the child.
2 All names are pseudonyms.

References

Arcia, E., Fernandez, M., Jaquez, M., 2004. Latina mothers' stances on stimulant medication: Complexity, conflict, and compromise. *J. Developmental Behav. Pediatrics 25* (5), 311–317.

Brinkman, W., Epstein, J., 2011. Promoting productive interactions between parents and physicians in the treatment of children with attention-deficit/hyperactivity disorder. *Expert. Rev. Neurotherapeutics 11* (4), 579–588.

Bussing, R., Faye, G., Mills, T., Garvan, C., 2007. Cultural variations in parental health benefits, knowledge, and information sources related to attention-deficit/hyperactivity disorder. *J. Family Issues 28*, 291–318.

Bussing, R., Koro-Ljungberg, M., Noguchi, K., Mason, D., Mayerson, G., Garvan, C., 2012. Willingness to use ADHD treatments: A mixed methods study of perceptions by adolescents, parents, health professionals and teachers. *Soc. Sci. Med. 74* (1), 92–100.

Costantino, G., Malgady, R., Primavera, L., 2009. Congruence between culturally competent treatment and cultural needs of older Latinos. *J. Consulting Clin. Psychol. 77* (5), 941–949.

Hansen, D., Hansen, E., 2006. Caught in a balancing act: Parents' dilemmas regarding their ADHD child's treatment with stimulant medication. *Qualitative Health Res. 16* (9), 1267–1285.

Hart, C., Kelleher, K., Drotar, D., Scholle, S., 2007. Parent-provider communication and parental satisfaction with care of children with psychosocial problems. *Patient Educ. Counseling 68*, 179–185.

Mikesell, L., Marti, F., Guzmán, J., McCreary, M., Zima, B., 2018. Affordances of mHealth technology and the structuring of clinic communication. *J. Appl. Commun. Res. 46* (3), 323–347.

Nobile, C., Drotar, D., 2003. Research on the quality of parent-provider communication in pediatric care: Implications and recommendations. *J. Developmental Behav. Pediatrics 24* (4), 279–290.

Ojeda, L., Flores, L., Meza, R., Morales, A., 2011. Culturally competent and qualitative research with Latino immigrants. *Hispanic J. Behav. Sci. 33* (2), 184–203.

Robinson, J., Tate, A., Heritage, J., 2016. Agenda-setting revisited: When and how do primary-care physicians solicit patients' additional concerns. *Patient Educ. Counseling 99* (5), 718–723.

Schoenthaler, A., Chaplin, W., Allegrante, J., Fernandez, S., Diaz-Gloster, M., Tobin, J., Ogedegbe, G., 2009. Provider communication effects medication adherence in hypertensive African Americans. *Patient Educ. Counseling 75*, 185–191.

Stivers, T., Barnes, R., 2017. Treatment recommendation actions, contingencies, and responses: An introduction. *Health Commun. 33* (11), 1331–1334.

Stivers, T., Heritage, J., Barnes, R., McCabe, R., Thompson, L., Toerien, M., 2018. Treatment recommendations as actions. *Health Commun. 33* (11), 1335–1344.

Tarn, D., Heritage, J., Paterniti, D., Hays, R., Kravitz, R., Wenger, N., 2006. Physician communication when prescribing new medications. *Arch. Intern. Med. 166*, 1855–1862.

Travell, C., Visser, J., 2006. "ADHD does bad stuff to you": Young people's and parents' experiences and perceptions of attention deficit hyperactivity disorder (ADHD). *Emotional Behavioural Difficulties 11* (3), 205–216.

Villalobos, B., Bridges, A., Anastasia, E., Ojeda, C., Rodriguez, J., Gomez, D., 2016. Effects of language concordance and interpreter use on therapeutic alliance in Spanish-speaking integrated behavioral health care patients. *Psychological Serv. 13* (1), 49–59.

Wissow, L., Brown, J., Krupnick, J., 2010. Therapeutic alliance in pediatric primary care: Preliminary evidence for a relationship with physician communication style and mothers' satisfaction. *J. Developmental Behav. Pediatrics 31* (2), 83–91.

Yeh, M., McCabe, K., Hough, R., Lau, A., Fakhry, F., Garland, A., 2005. Why bother with beliefs? Examining relationships between race/ethnicity, parental beliefs about causes of child problems, and mental health service use. *J. Consulting Clin. Psychol. 73* (5), 800–807.

Zima, B., Bussing, R., Tang, L., Zhang, L., Ettner, S., Belin, T., Wells, K., 2010. Quality of care for childhood ADHD in a large managed care Medicaid program. *J. Am. Acad. Child. Adolesc. Psychiatry 49* (12), 1225–1237.

Part II

Communication with adults

Chapter 8

Deception, fantasy and confabulation

What the stories of forensic patients with intellectual disabilities tell us about truth in therapeutic interactions

Sushie Jayne Dobbinson

Introduction

This chapter focuses on the qualitative analysis of interactions in which two patients with intellectual disabilities, Tommy and Billy, employ deception in the course of casual conversation in a clinical context. The patients are males in their 20s, detained in a medium secure psychiatric hospital in the UK. In the UK, this is termed a forensic setting, since patients are detained under sections of The Mental Health Act. The instances of deception have been selected to be both typical of the individuals and of the setting, in which varied forms of deception are frequently encountered. Despite its prevalence and the vast amount of literature devoted to it, in particular its detection, (e.g., DePaulo et al., 2003; DePaulo & Morris, 2004; Ekman, 2001; Feldman, Forrest, and Happ, 2002; Horvath, Jayne, and Buckley, 1994; Levine and Anders et al., 2000; Levine and Clare et al., 2014), the moment by moment construction of deception and how it works interactionally in a forensic context remain relatively unexplored (see also Drewett this volume).

In the forensic setting, where patients with a variety of presenting conditions are engaged in the difficult work of understanding and learning to manage a multitude of mental health conditions, understanding deception becomes an issue intimately related to recovery. The vast majority of the work of forensic hospitals is interactively constructed yet outside of particular theoretically specified therapy sessions, clinical practitioners rarely analyse the details of these interactions and so have little opportunity to understand the functions particular instances of deception may have for their patients. Indeed, training in interaction with patients is rarely explicit and generally limited to specific contexts where a therapy model is being followed, for example, Motivational Interviewing (Miller and Rollnick, 2013). Deception is generally understood to be a pathological feature of talk, and, particularly where it appears motiveless or flagrant can provoke strong adverse responses in interactants, who may fall back on lay responses, such as challenging or ignoring, without considering the impact this can have on therapeutic relationships or the psychosocial function of their patients. Since without the former, it is impossible to improve the latter, this seems to be a critical omission in forensic practice.

Using the qualitative methodology of conversation analysis (CA), this chapter examines two different types of deception and illustrates the type of insight a fine-grained analysis of talk can afford. This chapter argues that developing understanding of the role verbal deception has in interaction is of critical importance in understanding, engaging, and rehabilitating patients who frequently have recourse to it.

Three varieties of deception: Confabulation, pseudologia fantastica, and "common" deception

The literature on deceit and its detection is vast but tends to be skewed towards laboratory settings. DePaulo et al. published a comprehensive review on cues to deception which included 120 participant samples, yet almost none look at the details of interactions containing spontaneous deceptions (however, see Reynolds and Rendle-Short, 2011). Those that do tend to focus on high-stakes deception, for example, statements made in the context of criminal investigations (e.g., Horvath et al., 1994; Shaw, Porter, and ten Brinke, 2013). Most are concerned with detection of cues and favour methodologies in which deceptions are "placed", for example, in which participants are given instructions to lie. Such studies yield observable, countable data which allow for the presentation of concrete and provable findings. By contrast, the deceptions analysed here are mundane; they occur between interactants familiar with each other, in the ordinary course of conversation about nothing in particular, with no strongly motivating factor to deceive. There is no obvious reason for deception, and yet for both participants, it occurs often, regardless of audience and without any clear trigger. Indeed, its appearance is so pervasive as to suggest deception is intrinsic to the talk. The analyses presented suggest its most interesting meanings lie beyond surface structure and within the interactional context.

Confabulation

The invention of stories without purposeful intention to deceive, confabulation, is a feature of communication most often encountered within the brain-damaged population. Most usually associated with amnesic syndromes found in neuropsychological and psychiatric disorders such as dementia, this type of deceit is characterised not only by a lack of conscious intent to deceive but also an absence of obvious external motive, such as financial gain or escaping blame. Definitions of confabulation are various in the literature but generally include first, the notion of deviation from the truth and second, that deviation is contingent on memory problems.

Traditionally, confabulation is seen to have a locus within the internal psychological functioning, or more usually, dysfunction, of the individual. Orulv's (2006, p. 647) work with dementia patients, however, progresses this unitary view and examines confabulation from an interactional perspective, moving away from a personal, deficit-driven model to one which is socially situated and functionally driven. While it is certainly the case that confabulations are unintentionally false assertions or stories arising from biological pathology, Orulv points out their importance in the sense making processes of dementia patients. In her work, she analyses a story that two people with dementia make up together to make sense of a situation in which neither of them is sure what is happening. One tells the other that the people serving them tea are her guests and they are helping out, while in reality, they are both residents in a home and the guests are the staff. The paper demonstrates how the robustness of story-telling remains intact beyond the degeneration of memory and enables social identity to be preserved even as psychological and cognitive function decline. It elegantly illustrates why it helps people with intractable and degenerative memory loss if others enter their stories with them, rather than challenge or deny them. Such work as Orulv's has humanised the way we manage patients with this difficult and debilitating condition.

Pseudologia fantastica

Deception's most exotic manifestation is undoubtedly pseudologia fantastica (PF) also known as mythomania or pathological lying, first described in the literature in 1891 by the German psychiatrist, Anton Delbruck, around the same time that confabulation was first described. PF is a sub-clinical condition which has mainly been of interest as a feature of Munchausen's syndrome, or factitious disorder, a phenomenon first labelled by Asher, which has illness-based fantastical story telling as its core symptom. People with factitious disorder neither seek extrinsic gain from their falsifications nor are they deluded or psychotic. Asher describes a type of patient well known to medical staff, who frequents hospitals feigning symptoms, ostensibly to seek treatment but who often then discharges him or herself against advice. These patients travel from hospital to hospital, often getting into conflicts with staff or becoming unreasonably litigious. They recount an "immediate history which is always acute and harrowing yet not entirely convincing" (p 339). The lies they tell are described as being out of proportion with the apparent aim (to receive treatment) in both extent and content and are told to almost everyone encountered. Exotic personal histories, such as being in the Special Air Service, experiencing torture or working as a spy are often included. The stories tend to contain elements of truth; the patient may in fact be having or have suffered serious illness and have scars which add "artistic validity" to their accounts (p. 339).

Stripped of its medicalised context, PF is certainly recognizable to most people. We have all encountered someone who tells lies for no apparent reason, which are easily recognisable as untrue. Sometimes the lies themselves are extravagant or florid, but often it is the sheer number of stories over time that rings false. The poor response such tales elicit does not seem to deter the telling of them nor is it clear what motivates the teller since there is no obvious gain to be had. At their worst, such stories can cause serious social and even physical harm to others for example, if they involve false allegations. Importantly, in the clinical context, it can be hard to know how to respond to them without provoking conflict.

PF is not a diagnosable condition but is nevertheless an identifiable phenomenon which has the features listed below.

- The fluent and habitual telling of stories which mix truth and deception. The stories can have any theme, but the teller is usually the central character and often portrayed as hero or victim
- Onset in adolescence
- A lack of control in the frequency and context of the story-telling. The stories appear to derive from a compulsive desire to include them in interactive dialogue. They are not demanded from the context, as for example, a false account of events presented in order to explain, excuse, or discount socially deviant behaviour may be
- There does not appear to be any underpinning, externally obvious motive of profit or gain, for example, financial or sexual advantage or improvement in physical well-being
- If challenged, the PF story-teller may admit their deception or change story, and so differ from schizophrenics whose delusional beliefs are fixed in nature and resistant to reasoning (King and Ford, 1988; Newmark, Adityanjee, and Kay, 1999).

Outside of the context of factitious disorder, PF prevalence has scarcely been researched. However, based on data from 1915, a prevalence of around 1% within the forensic population is estimated, similar to that of factitious disorder within the general population.

Common deception

Most of the studies which provide the evidence for ordinary deception involve lies which have been placed within a participant's repertoire under laboratory conditions. Deception detection is a fiendishly complex business which must take context into account and cannot be reduced to a simple list of features. However, DePaulo's work points to some fairly robust tendencies that regularly recur across studies. Ordinary lies tend to make less sense, are less logical and less plausible than truthful statements. When lying, people are more distant, impersonal, evasive and unclear, and offer fewer details. They seem to talk less, using fewer words rather than taking up less floor time, suggesting more hesitation and less semantic content. A small number of studies suggests that liars make more negative statements and complaints.

The two tales of Tommy and Billy: A fantastical slap vs an ordinary loss

Tommy and Billy have both committed serious interpersonal offences and been the victims of offences, a not uncommon profile in forensic intellectual disability (FLD) communities. In comparison with ward peers, both are at the higher end of verbal ability.

At the time of the recordings, Tommy was in his late 20s and had been resident in secure care since his teens. Prior to this, Tommy also spent many years resident in children's homes. His receptive verbal age equivalent score is 15. Practitioners often remark on Tommy's frequent use of deception noting a tendency towards grandiosity and that he appears unable to form attachments with peers. Tommy has been diagnosed with narcissistic and anti-social personality disorder as well as his intellectual disability.

Billy was in his early 20s at the time of the study and although had only recently come into secure care had a long history of offending. Like Tommy, Billy had a difficult early childhood involving many care placements. His verbal age equivalent score is 12 years. Billy struggles with accepting responsibility for his offences and expresses little empathy with the victims of his offending. His psychological reports describe him as a fragile narcissist.

Tommy

Extract 1 has been taken from a conversation between S (the author) and Tommy in which Tommy tells S about how he got into trouble with a girl at a football game. Tommy's deception is at line 3, *I got slapped*, inserted into the dialogue as an interruption of S as she attempts to give Tommy positive feedback about his football successes (Tommy's escorts at the game confirmed that while he talked briefly to Lorraine, no slapping took place).

Extract 1

```
S    (.) hats bri^lliant (0.6) thạts
     what you wanna 'h[hear isn't it]
T                    [I got slapped]
S    (0.3) 'who slạ pped you
T    Lorràine hh bubbling,suppressed laugh
S    'what fŏ r
T    .hh hh I 'WAlked up to her n went 'all rI ^ght
```

```
         Lor´raine n she went huh.hhh ↓WHY uv you been
         to JV for a while gruff
T        n I went (0.1) ´well its ´cos (.) we ant had
         the ´staff to còme.hhh n she went (0.2) ↓´well
         (0.2) im na (.)nnòyed wi yer (0.1) gruff
T        n then she i̯ t me n I went ↑O::WW:.hhh n
         ´thEnn (0.2) I WA̯lked ´off ´went n ´talked to
         Pàt ´whos er ´mum (0.4) n said ´ello to er n
         then Lo- n walked back to Lo´rraine n she
         sla̯pped me a´gain n I went ↑what was thât
         one for.hh n she went ʹTHAts forʹmissing me
         bI:rthday yerʹbegg.hhar hh.Hh I s.hHai.h d
                oh IʹcA:n´t ↑wI̧n wi you cÀn I
S (0.3) t.´is Lorr´aine from:
```

In the conversation from which the extract is taken, of which just two lines are shown here (lines 1–2), S is mainly occupied with housekeeping the talk, seeking information by asking questions and clarifications (repairs), making background supportive comments, or evaluating Tommy's contributions, the latter always positively. Conversely, giving information and telling stories form the basis of Tommy's much longer turns, accounting for 81% of the words spoken (1025 Tommy words versus 238 S words). Incongruent to what might be expected given S's highly facilitative style, 27% of Tommy's turns interrupt or overlap S (by comparison, just 2% of S turns overlap or interrupt Tommy). Lines 1–3 in Extract 1 are an example of a typical interruption, here of an S positive evaluation. Overlaps at the end of another's turn can be relatively benign. However, in this context, in which positive evaluations and supportive comments are overlapped so pervasively, the impression is rather of hostility, suggesting a marked lack of orientation to other. Indeed, Tommy's clinicians confirm they experience conversation with him as rejecting and frustrating saying *he never listens.*

By introducing the slap story with its crux (also its abstract), Tommy positions it for greatest impact. Importantly, *I got slapped* is grammatically passive, which allows Tommy to avoid mentioning the identity of the agent-performer of the slapping. Because of this missing information, Tommy effectively forces, or "projects" to use the CA term, S's next turn as a "repair request" (request for clarification), which S obligingly provides in line 4. Tommy's one-word response, *Lorraine*, line 5, marked by suppressed laughter, high starting pitch and bubbling voice quality, suggests emotional investment in the content. Tommy sounds delighted. Tommy has also repeated an earlier strategy of giving a one-word answer which omits crucial information, so projecting another S repair request at line 6, *what for.* The device of withholding information steers S to ask questions, and so invites her collusion in topicalizing the story behind the slap. The work Tommy puts into ensuring the involvement of S as well as his engagement with its content indicate that this is an important story for him.

The story body is just as well-structured. The complicating action is constructed as a single, rapid, uninterruptable sequence, with no pauses for S interruptions (the 0.4-second pause at line 16 is in the middle of an incomplete grammar and tone unit, hence unlikely to be taken as an opportunity to interrupt). Tommy's story includes eight *went* structures, which lend the story-sequence rhythm and cohesion through lexical repetition. Phonetically, word initial /w/ occurs 21 times in the 111-word sequence between lines 14 and 21, a poetic device similar to alliteration called "andiplosis" in the context of conversation (Wooffit and Holt, 2011). Further evidence of Tommy's flair for poetic cohesion is seen at the finale, line 21, *oh I can't win wi you can I.* This is chiasmus, a type of structural reversal.

Poetic devices in everyday talk can indicate an introspective focus on internal mental imagery, which would be consistent with the lack of concern towards interlocutor demonstrated by Tommy's interruptions and overlaps.

The prosodic patterning in Tommy's narrative augments the phonetic cohesion. Tommy begins his story with relatively narrow pitch movements which become increasingly wide as the story approaches its crux, is followed by a shallower movement for *what was that for*, before moving into the final section *that's for missing me birthday yer beggar* which has the widest and most complex pitch movement of all, consisting of two closely tied pitch peaks. This prosodic patterning not only animates the story, but gives it audible structure.

Finally, Tommy voices his story's characters, although does so inconsistently with their gender. Lorraine is gruff and deep, while Tommy voices himself as neutral in pitch and tone. Lorraine's reported speech is angry and abrupt, while Tommy presents himself as calm and reasonable. Speaking as Lorraine, Tommy expresses frustration and anger at his not being able to attend football games and letting down his friends. The device of voicing allows him, at the same time as expressing anger, to present himself as a voice of reason.

That this story is the product of mental rehearsal is, then, evident at multiple levels. This, as well as the content portrayal of himself as both hero and victim, the character around which the action turns, and the way in which Tommy uses S to help him insert the story into the dialogue rather than it's being demanded from context, are all features of PF.

Billy

In Extract 2 below, Billy answers my question about how he came to be on the ward where the conversation takes place. Billy's tendency to evasiveness in the context of difficult topics appears straight away as he constructs his explanation of being in prison as arising from the loss of his house rather than due to the commission of an offence.

Extract 2

B I was actually in 'Lynn Pri̠ son for a 'month in re'mand

S (0.1) ri ̀ght (.) OK

B thiss were 'throu::gh (.) because I 'losss (0.4) a 'pla::ce
 (0.2) >inWạ ssily< (.) > I lost house<

S (0.3) you 'lost a 'house in Wạ ssily

B yeàh >cos oviously it were re̠ nted < n:: (0.7) it were:: (0.2)
 'under (0.1) cà:re (0.4)

S OK̀ =

B ='package n (0.4) >oviously I were managed to it n:: (0.8) so
 many warns that I had n:: <(0.1) I got chụ cked out

S (0.2) t. ÒK

B so I 'lost the 'ouse (.) 'pfrough 'that

S (0.3) was it a hou- a 'place you had on your o^:wn

B it 'was ye̠ a:h it was a (.) thre̠ e bedroomed house 'rented (0.2)
 °n° (.)>there wạ s another lad lived there °buv° < (0.1) wa-
 (0.3) e got 'chucked out before I̠: did

S (0.2) OK̠

B (0.4) sa::h (0.2) then it were just me on me ọ::wn (0.4) but
 managed to get me chucked ọut (.) as well so:::

S (0.4) OK wa- di- what ↑hâppened

B (0.2) t. wha it wạ s I came in one- (.) one 'nights I came in quite
 late n I didnt me̠an ter: (0.1) cos oviously the 'rules were
 (0.1) meant to be in before te̠n (1.2) annd (.) came in quite lạ
 te nn (0.6) nọ it was a we̠ekend (0.1) so I 'came in before ele-
 (0.1) ele̠ ven (0.7) or twe̠lve n: she said o-:h ri̠ ::ght (0.3)
 yeah she wụ nt 'appy (.) 'carer wasnt she were what ti⁻mes this
 °n so m said° (0.4) look >Im sorry< I was bi̠ king back n:: (0.7)
 {sniff} t.uh '>tried to get back ↑ọme <{clears throat} next
 da^y:: (.) I got a le̠ tter 'frough (.) saying Ive had muh 'third
 written 'warning which was.hhh (0.5) I were getting 'kicked out
 n I >would have to find < another 'plac::e (.) to li̠ ve (1.0)

As with Tommy, Billy's story has a conventional narrative structure; abstract, complicating action, and coda are all present, but, unlike Tommy's story, poetic devices are not. Further, Billy's story is markedly less fluent than Tommy's and contains a large amount of hesitations and reformulations, as such suggestive of an absence of rehearsal. His prosody is much flatter with none of the variability of Tommy's, giving an authoritative tone. Much of it is delivered fast and with low volume.

While Tommy boldly places the deceit, *I got slapped* as abstract, Billy's deceptions occur as more subtle tracings within the narrative. For example, in lines 3–4, Billy volunteers the information about losing his house in Wassily, seeming to own up to his responsibility for losing it. However, his use of *obviously* (rendered as *oviously*) at lines 6, 9, and 24 suggests something different. *Obviously* here works like *of course* as a "negative politeness pragmatic particle", that is, common knowledge among those "in the know", and which is covertly authoritative in the context of the interaction. This device in this context effectively allows Billy to align with the authorities. Billy sounds as if he is assessing the behaviour of someone else, since the expectations are *obvious* to him.

Later at lines 19–20, Billy doesn't quite own up to responsibility again, this time using grammar. At line 16–17, he mentions the *other lad* who *got chucked out* before him. Two lines later, the passive with subject pronoun omitted (*managed to get me chucked out as well*) implies that *the other lad* was somehow responsible for Billy's unravelling, despite, given the reported sequence of events, this not being logically possible. Billy's passive is not quite the same as Tommy's, since Tommy's was grammatically complete. Here Billy elides *he*, a referential element that might be expected in the context. Oh (2006) notes this device allows speakers to avoid making a choice between referents, usefully here for Billy to sidestep his commitment and instead introduce ambiguity about whose fault it was that he got chucked out.

Evasiveness in the form of hesitations, dysfluencies, incomplete explanations, and events that do not match up are all present in the story's complicating action between lines 22 and 40 and accord with De Paulo's findings that deceptions appear as less logical, less plausible and as unclear, evasive distant, impersonal and lacking in detail. For example, at line 24, Billy tells me that he had to be in before ten, but was late, then at line 26 he says he came in before the curfew, although is not clear whether this was eleven or twelve o'clock. It is difficult to locate deception since it has almost no lexical locus. Tucked within dysfluent incompletions, missing antecedents, internal inconsistency, and some subtle uses of grammar, Billy's deception is committed as much through omission as assertion, with none of the rehearsed feel of Tommy's.

Relevance to practice: The truths beneath the deceptions

By using hostile overlaps, passives, and minimal responses, Tommy orchestrates the conversation to a point where he can deliver his story. The story itself includes a great deal of rehearsed detail, as well as voicings, use of tone, grammar, and poetic devices. As a stand-alone piece, it would not look out of place in a soap opera or play.

On the other hand, Billy's story, filled with hesitations and dysfluencies, is clearly spontaneous. The deceptions lie in what Billy doesn't say as much as what he does. He aligns himself with an authoritative perspective and implies, but avoids stating, that his unravelling was someone else's responsibility. When he provides details, they are confusing and inconsistent:

"innuendo, strategic ambiguity, and crucial omissions allow the misinformer to profit from lies without, technically, telling any".

The difference is mirrored by behaviour; Tommy loves to perform, while Billy strenuously resists the spotlight. Billy seems to have adopted a strategy of mystification: by maintaining social distance, he seeks to control his contacts, and, through evasiveness, omission, and a presentation of un-remarkableness in speech, what others are able to perceive of him (Goffman, 1990, p. 74).

Tommy's poetic devices suggest inwardly focused motivation and his narrative, while superficially engaging, in fact displaces alignment to con-versational partner in favour of alignment to his own internal dialogue. Interestingly, during a post data-collection reflection session, Tommy stated that his most abiding experience of conversation was that *no one ever listens to me*. His story is, then, told perhaps less with his listener in mind, but more as a primarily expressive act arising from Tommy's own internal mental state. Meanwhile, Billy's story orients more to the listener as a representative of an authority to whom issues of guilt and blame are a primary concern. Perhaps due to his lengthier detention, Tommy's story speaks of immersion in his internal world, while Billy's orients towards the understandings that dominate forensic settings.

Reflection: Fitting deception into practice

Where it takes place regularly in the repertoire of a speaker, PF can cause all sorts of problems within the community as well as in the forensic context. While some FLD patients are naïve in their honesty, some on the ward from which the extracts are taken mark nearly every extended interaction with false material. Including Tommy, at the time of writing three out of eight regularly used PF. Clinicians may feel unable to establish a bond of trust while peers may be driven to ostracise their fantastically inclined co-residents, with the potential to cause serious rifts in ward dynamics. The clinical literature offers little advice in how best to deal with it, other than to refer for psychoanalysis; an expensive, time-consuming, and largely in-accessible treatment for FLD patients due to the cognitive and linguistic demands required.

The lack of a diagnostic category for PF means that forensic mental health workers who may frequently encounter the behaviour are unable to find little systematic research on the topic. The sparse availability of com-munication specialists in forensic settings further inhibits understanding. Thus, a perfect storm is created. Poor understanding of deception leads to the practise of ignoring, dismissing, or addressing it in ways that damage, increasing the likelihood that it will be used by the patients who continue to feel as if they are not listened to, perhaps embedding that experience in evermore florid tales.

If examined in context, however, deception can be a rich source of information about a patient, their internal mental state and psychosocial functioning. When the findings around Tommy's fantastical story telling were shared with the clinical team, a difference in approach percolated slowly through the ward. A change in terminology was normalized, in which talk was of patients confabulating rather than lying. The distinction was also mobilised to differentiate the stories told by patients with delusions and gave teams a different way of thinking about non-factual stories beyond use of the term "psychotic", a word which can sometimes be used misleadingly in psychiatric contexts.

Unfortunately, by the time the work was done, the relationship between Tommy and staff had become exhausted. Tommy was keen to move on and start again elsewhere. Before he went, an attempt was made to interest him in channelling his story-telling skills by writing for the hospital magazine. He gave himself a persona as football expert, work I think he enjoyed. With more time we could perhaps have given him the opportunity to develop this side of himself.

Newmark and Kay suggest PF should be conceptualized as a disorder of the self; there is an inability to "regulate or moderate … sense of self and self-esteem" giving rise to grandiosity as a response to "profound feelings of unworthiness, emptiness and alienation" (p. 93). This evokes Orulv's memory-impaired interactants using confabulation to formulate or maintain identity. While PF does not derive from memory impairment, the lack of control over the behaviour and its persistent nature, suggests it tells an equally functional story.

Orulv's story-telling dementia patients are falling back on a mechanism more robust than memory: story-telling allows them to navigate whatever world presents itself to them. Similarly, the two very different narratives of Tommy and Billy tell how the world looks from where they are, and how they seek to escape from it. In their deceptions, we see both patients attempting to create selves that fit. Tommy projects a world where he is popular and socially valued, while Billy tries to find a world where his mistakes have an innocent cause. Tommy's anger, Billy's confusion, expressed beyond the words, within structures, tones, and other devices, weave a second story into the narrative.

Conclusion

FLD patients often have chaotic personal histories and, while detained for their own criminal activity, have often been subject to victimisation themselves. For anyone with an LD, engaging with the criminal justice system is likely to be at best confusing and at worst unremittingly disempowering. Struggling to accept past experiences, that offer few positives in terms of self image and little in the way of consistent narrative in which to situate those experiences, to some extent represents a similar background to that of

---

Box 8.1   Practical tips

Practical tips for communication

- When most people hear a fantastical tale, they hesitate, then focus on moving the talk on by asking questions with no direct relevance to the story (as I do in Extract 1 line 22) which can feel rejecting to the patient. Try responding to the emotional thread of the story instead, saying something like "I hate missing someone's birthday".
- Explore creative strategies with FLD patients, addressing the experience of feeling as if they are not listened to by facilitating opportunities to express themselves. This could involve the use of art, music, sport, or story-telling.
- Use self-esteem work as a matter of course with any patients who frequently use deception, working on building their sense of identity.

---

acquired memory impairment. In both cases, the individual struggling to make sense of present self and experience, draws from a limited resource of meaning-rich past selves and experience.

When viewed as an emergent product of interaction rather than as an individual choice about behaviour, FLD deception begins to look more like a resilience-enabling strategy rather than an intrinsically divisive or controlling behaviour. Crucially, practitioners are more likely to feel able to engage with deception when viewed this way, thus opening up a route for therapeutic intervention. To conclude, and based on the analysis in this chapter, I offer some practical tips for communication in Box 8.1.

References

DePaulo, B., Lindsay, J.J., Malone, B.E., Muhlenbruck, L., Charlton, K., Cooper, H., 2003. Cues to deception. *Psychol. Bullet. 129*, 74–118.

DePaulo, B.M., Morris, W.L., 2004. Discerning lies from truths: behavioural cues to deception and the indirect pathway of intuition. In: Granhag, P.A., Stromwall, L.A. (Eds.), *The Detection of Deception in Forensic Contexts.* Cambridge University Press, Cambridge, pp. 15–40.

Ekman, P., 2001. *Lies: Clues to Deceit in the Marketplace, Politics and Marriage.* WW Norton and Company Inc., New York.

Feldman, R., Forrest, J., Happ, B., 2002. Self-presentation and verbal deception: Do self presenters lie more. *Basic Appl. Soc. Psychol. 24* (2), 163–170.

Goffman, E., 1981. Footing. In: Goffman, E. (Ed.), *Forms of Talk*. University of Pennsylvania Press, Philadelphia, PA, pp. 124–159.

Goffman, E., 1990. *The Presentation of Self in Everyday Life*. Penguin, London.

Horvath, F., Jayne, B., Buckley, J., 1994. Differentiation of truthful and deceptive criminal suspects in behaviour analysis interviews. *J. of Forensic Sciences 39*, 793–807.

King, B., Ford, C.V., 1988. Pseudologia fantastica. *Aacta Psychiatrica Scandinavia 77* (1), 6.

Levine, T., Anders, L., Banas, J., Baum, K., Endo, K., Hu, A., Wong, N., 2000. Norms, expectations, and deception: A norm violation model of veracity judgements. *Communication Monographs 67* (2). doi:10.1080/03637750009376500.

Levine, T., Clare, D., Green, T., Serota, K., Park, H., 2014. The effects of truth-lie base rate on interactive deception detection accuracy. *Hum. Commun. Res. 40*, 350–372.

Miller, W., Rollnick, S., 2013. *Motivational Interviewing: Helping People Change*. The Guilford Press, New York.

Newmark, N., Adityanjee, Kay, J., 1999. Pseudologia and factitious disorder: review of the literature and a case report. *Compr. Psychiatry 40* (2), 89–95.

Oh, S.-Y., 2006. English zero anaphora as an interactional resource II. *Discourse Stud. 8* (6), 817–846.

Orulv, L., Hyden, L.-C., 2006. Confabulation: Sense-making, self-making and world-making in dementia. *Discourse Stud. 85* (5), 647–673.

Reynolds, E., Rendle-Short, J., 2011. Cues to deception in context: Response latency/gaps in denials and blame shifting. *Br. J. Soc. Psychol. 50*, 431–449.

Shaw, J., Porter, S., ten Brinke, L., 2013. Catching liars: Training mental health and legal professionals to detect high-stakes lies. *J. Forensic. Psychiatry. Psychol. 24* (2), 145–159.

Wooffit, R., Holt, N., 2011. Introspective discourse and the poetics of subjective experience. *Res. Lang. Soc. Interact. 44* (2), 135–156.

Chapter 9

Communicating about feelings

Examples from depression care

Brandon C. Yarns and Elizabeth Bromley

Introduction

Understanding patients' feelings is important to providing high-quality mental healthcare (see Farrelly, this volume, for discussion of the power of words). For instance, making accurate diagnoses of patients' emotional problems using the *Diagnostic and Statistical Manual of Mental Disorders* (*DSM-5*) relies on understanding patients' feelings and categorizing them into certain diagnostic categories (American Psychiatric Association, 2013). The consequences of undiagnosed and untreated emotional problems are well known to impact negatively physical health, quality of life, and functioning (Moussavi et al., 2007; Wrenn et al., 2013).

Mental health professionals often wish to elicit patients' healthy, adaptive feelings to encourage positive mental health. Certain emotions, such as anger, sadness, joy, surprise, disgust, and fear have been described as determined by evolution (Panksepp, 1998) and universal across people from different cultural backgrounds (Ekman and Friesen, 1971). Such emotions are thought to be important because they help people make choices and provide us with information from within about what to *do* in certain situations (Panksepp, 1998; Scherer, 2005). For instance, healthy guilt is thought to promote repair after one has done wrong, and some have suggested that anger can be health-promoting when it results in assertiveness and the establishment of healthy boundaries (Panksepp, 1998; Vaillant, 1997). Finally, healthy emotions may add richness and fullness to life. The late psychotherapist, researcher, and author Leigh McCullough Vaillant wrote, "The more one can laugh when happy, cry when sad, use anger to set firm limits, make love passionately, and give and receive tenderness fully and openly, the further one is from suffering" (Vaillant, 1997). Therefore, it is essential for mental health professionals to strive to understand our patients' communications about their feelings.

Yet in the mental health clinic, patients often have difficulty articulating their feelings in response to direct questions, providing complex, indirect, or ambivalent responses instead (Bromley et al., 2016; Yarns et al., 2018). If mental health professionals are not able to make sense of patients' communications about their feelings, they could be left baffled and unable to make accurate diagnoses and treatment plans or provide support for patients' healthy, adaptive emotions.

The most common methods used to understand patients' feelings – both to diagnose emotional problems and identify the presence of healthy, adaptive feelings – in the clinical setting rely on eliciting patients' self-report of their feelings, either by asking patients direct questions about feelings in clinical interviews or, increasingly, by using self-report screening checklists and questionnaires (Kroenke, Spitzer, and Williams, 2001, 2003; Spitzer et al., 2006; Yarns et al., 2018). Yet it is well-recognized that there are limitations to relying on patients' self-reports of feelings elicited either by symptom checklists or in the clinical interview. For instance, prior research has highlighted the limitations of screening self-report checklists and questionnaires, which are limited by numerical thresholds and may not be effective at diagnosing emotional problems in all populations (Barrett et al., 1988; Borowsky et al., 2000). Therefore, new clinical tools are necessary to elicit, distinguish, and characterize feelings that may be insufficiently articulated or entirely unspoken.

Using interview data from Partners in Care (PIC), a multicenter randomized-controlled trial of quality improvement for depression (Rubenstein et al., 1999; Schoenbaum et al., 2001; Sherbourne et al., 2001; Wells, 1999; Wells et al., 2000; Wells, Sherbourne, Schoenbaum, and Ettner et al., 2004), we provide examples of the complex and often baffling responses patients provide in response to direct questions. To make sense of these responses, we propose a new method of clinical listening that relies on listening for patterns of verbal expression of feelings. Our method involves listening for three qualitatively different categories of words patients use to describe their feelings – specific feeling words, vague feeling words, and physical words. We derived these three categories of words using content analysis of semi-structured interviews collected to evaluate long-term depression outcomes among PIC participants. We provide examples of each category from these data and describe the theoretical and empirical justification for the three categories to help clinicians learn to listen for patterns of feeling words. We then demonstrate how eliciting specific feeling words provides more actionable information for the mental health clinician than either vague feeling words or physical words. Finally, we provide suggestions for techniques clinicians can use to elicit specific feeling words that derive from our data and our own clinical experience.

Difficulties in communicating about feelings: Context and Literature Review

Clinicians have observed that patients often have difficulty articulating their feelings (Freud A., 1966; Freud S., 1936). We have similarly observed this common yet peculiar phenomenon in our own clinical practice. Indeed, we have come to expect that patients will struggle to articulate their feelings when they need help with them. Especially in the brief patient interviews that are characteristic of current clinical practice, patients' most meaningful and profound emotional experiences are often undeclared or unspoken.

What makes it so difficult for mental health patients to communicate their feelings? Several theories have been put forward. The psychodynamic tradition has been particularly focused on this phenomenon. Freud's eventual understanding of this phenomenon was expressed in his Second Theory of Anxiety. Freud asserted that anxiety is a signal that any thought, feeling, or fantasy that threatens bonds with caretakers becomes dangerous and is to be avoided. The avoidance manifests as defenses which distort and distance the patient from dangerous feelings and can adversely impact the ability of the patient to recall and directly communicate such feelings (Freud, 1936).

Later, Sifneos and colleagues (1977) developed the concept of alexithymia, which refers to patients' difficulties with identifying and describing their feelings, as well as externally-oriented thinking and a limited imaginal capacity (Bagby, Parker, and Taylor, 1994). Alexithymia can be assessed using a 20-item self-report measure, the Toronto Alexithymia Scale-20 item (TAS-20) (Bagby et al., 1994). Higher levels of alexithymia, as assessed with the TAS-20, have been associated with several adverse health outcomes, especially post-traumatic stress disorder (Frewen et al., 2008) and chronic pain (Lumley et al., 2011). However, many studies do not show robust correlations between alexithymia and health outcomes (Kojima, 2012; Lane et al., 2015). Some have asserted the lack of strong associations between alexithymia and health outcomes may also be a problem with patients' self-report: Is someone who has difficulty identifying and describing their feelings aware of such difficulties and thus able to accurately report them on a questionnaire (Lane et al., 2015)?

Other constructs have been developed to assess patients' overall comfort with emotional experience and expression, deriving from different theoretical traditions outside of psychodynamic theory. For instance, the concept of experiential avoidance, which derives from learning theory (e.g., classical and operant conditioning) and acceptance and commitment therapy (Hayes, Strosahl, and Wilson, 1999), describes attempts to avoid thoughts, feelings, memories, physical sensations, and other experiences, even when this avoidance creates harm in the long-run (Hayes et al., 1996). Even while positing no unconscious conflict that motivates avoidance of negative emotions, experiential avoidance also emphasizes that avoidance of negative emotions can be detrimental to health and functioning (Hayes et al., 1996). A self-report measure has also been developed to assess experiential avoidance, and, similar to alexithymia, this measure demonstrates some associations to health outcomes (Fledderus, Bohlmeijer, and Pieterse, 2010).

Other similar constructs that refer to psychological difficulties with emotional experience or expression come from other theoretical and empirical work. These include ambivalence over emotional expression (King and Emmons, 1990), affect control (Williams, Chambless, and Ahrens, 1997), affect phobia (McCullough, 2003), and conflicted emotions (Bhatia et al., 2009). Each of these concepts implies some psychological discomfort with emotions or emotional expression (e.g., ambivalence, need to control, or fear of emotions).

Still others suggest that certain populations may have more difficulty with communicating their emotions than others due to dispositional or cultural differences, rather than psychological factors. For instance, some research suggests that men and women may communicate differently about their feelings, and that men may be less likely to discuss their feelings openly (Borowsky et al., 2000; DeSteno, Gross, and Kubzansky, 2013; Else-Quest et al., 2012). African Americans and Hispanics may also be less likely to openly discuss their feelings (Borowsky et al., 2000). Indeed, a large cross-cultural literature identifies significant variability in the experience and expression of low mood (DeSteno et al., 2013; Kirmayer 1989). Other researchers have posited that developmental experiences and processes of socialisation may alter individuals' capacity to express emotion (Briggs, 1970; Capps and Ochs, 1995; Shapiro, 2011).

Mental health patients often come to treatment distressed, and patients who are in distress can have more difficulty clearly articulating their distress, particularly when it is characterized by a great deal of anxiety that can interrupt their ability to think clearly and communicate effectively. Short-term dynamic psychotherapy models, among others, point to a clinical need for regulation of excessive distress to promote clear communication from patients about their feelings (Davanloo, 1990; McCullough, 2003).

Whether due to psychological conflicts about emotional experience and expression, cultural or dispositional differences, or distress, the difficulties patients have in communicating their feelings in the clinical interview are well-documented in the literature. In the next section, we go on to report additional examples of this phenomenon from our research.

Examples of difficulties communicating about feelings from research

We have previously reported in detail on the complex statements one research interview respondent used to describe her feelings (Yarns et al., 2018). The following examples of patients' difficulties in articulating feelings derive from four respondents to semi-structured interviews conducted as part of Partners in Care (PIC), a randomized-controlled trial of quality improvement for depression in 46 managed care clinics across the United States (Rubenstein et al., 1999; Schoenbaum et al., 2001; Sherbourne et al., 2001; Wells, 1999; Wells et al., 2000; Wells et al., 2004). At enrollment, all PIC participants reporting depressive symptoms on a structured instrument were randomized to a control or intervention group. Then, participants completed surveys on depressive symptoms and other factors every 6 months for 2 years then at 5- and 9-year follow-up time points. At the 10-year follow-up time point, a subsample was invited to participate in up to three semi-structured interviews over approximately three months about their illness experience. Interviews at the 10-year follow-up time point consisted of open-ended questions followed by probes that focused on the subjective experience of living with depression and the long-term effects of the study's quality improvement interventions. Interviewers were trained for the study, and some interviewers also had clinical experience. A total of 280 respondents completed at least one interview, which was audio recorded. These interviews were of interest to us because the probes in each area contained specific questions about the respondents' feelings.

We used purposive sampling to identify respondents who were likely to provide complex examples of their emotional experiences: respondents age 65 years and older with chronic depression, which was defined as scoring depressed on all depression screening checklists (i.e., every 6 months for 2 years then at 5- and 9-year follow-up time points). We identified five respondents who met these criteria, but one was excluded because there was only one interview, which did not provide enough examples of emotional experience. Our final sample included four respondents with three interviews. Audio recorded interviews were professionally transcribed. The Institutional Review Board (IRB) at the RAND Corporation approved the PIC study, acquisition of the PIC 10-year follow-up interviews, and our new analysis.

Across the four respondents' interviews, 58 examples of probes for feelings were located. Most often this included questions such as, "How do you feel?" or "How did that make you feel?" Respondents' answers to these questions were often quite complex. We found only nine of the 58 examples in which respondents answered a question about how they felt with a response that referred to a specific feeling. Here is an example:

```
Interviewer (I): How does that make you feel that you can't
                 be there?
Respondent (R): I feel so sad, so sad.
```

In this example, the respondent was clearly able to communicate that she was sad about the situation under discussion. If this exchange were to occur in the mental health treatment setting, the respondent's clear communication of sadness – along with other cues such as nonverbal communication – could help the mental health professional understand that this patient needed help with her grieving and healing her sadness. Specific interventions could then be provided to allow space to explore her grief and heal it, and mental health diagnoses and unnecessary treatments could possibly be avoided.

More often, however, respondents answered questions about how they were feeling with far more complex responses. For 49 of the 58 answers to questions about how they were feeling, respondents did not answer with any clear communication about how they were feeling. In the following example, the respondent does not mention any specific feelings:

I: And emotionally, how do you feel the next day after a night like that?

R: Pretty *bad*. I'm not getting anything done. I don't have that much long left to go, and I've got a lot of stuff. It just piles up and piles up, stuff that I need to do, and I can't do it because I'm too *tired* to do it, because I can't sleep at night. Like last night, I didn't finally fall asleep until – I don't know – five or six o'clock, and then I sleep all day, and I'm not getting anything done. And even when I get up, I'm still *tired* and *worn out*. [italics added]

Despite the interviewer specifying that she was asking how the respondent felt *emotionally*, instead the respondent used a vague phrase, "pretty bad", and then redirected her attention toward her external circumstances, "stuff … just piles up and piles up", and her physical symptoms, feeling "tired" and "worn out". For this latter respondent, these communications which relied on reporting vague and physical symptoms, rather than specific feelings, may have had treatment implications. Based on other parts of the interview, we were able to determine that she was not taking psychiatric medications or in psychotherapy at the time of these interviews. However, she was taking opioid medications for physical pain.

In other examples, respondents did not describe their experience at all. Instead, they replied with thoughts or other statements that did not answer the question directly or shed any light on what they were feeling, as seen below:

I: How does that make you feel emotionally, feeling worn out all month and having everything hurt?

R: I think, I guess that this can't go on like this.

In this example, the interviewer struggles to make an important distinction between the respondent's emotional experience and physical experience. She asks what the respondent felt *emotionally* about her physical symptoms of fatigue and pain. However, the respondent replied with a thought rather than any words to describe her emotional experience.

Evidence-based practice: Using patterns of verbal expression of feelings in the mental health setting

Based on our literature review and the complex and unique answers respondents provided to questions about how they were feeling, academic and experienced community reviewers from different cultural backgrounds reviewed transcripts, collaborated to develop coding categories, and then coded interviews to develop a technique for an improved understanding of how respondents were communicating about their feelings. The goal of this technique was to analyse the often-confusing communications patients provide when asked about their feelings in order to identify patterns of language use that may suggest strategies to elicit meaningful and actionable information in the clinical setting.

To that end, we identified three categories of words that respondents used to describe their experience: *specific feeling words*, *vague feeling words*, and *physical words*. For research purposes, we counted the words in each category of word and calculated category word per 100 words spoken by the respondent, which allowed for comparisons of word use across different respondents and different interviews that contained different numbers of overall word counts (Cowie et al., 2001). All members of the research team were involved in developing definitions for the codes and distinguishing one category from another. Table 9.1 summarizes the word categories and provides examples of each. Below, we describe each of the categories in detail.

Specific feeling words

Specific feeling words were defined as words used by respondents to describe one discrete emotional experience that had occurred in the past or during the interview. Examples of specific feeling words included: *happy*, *sad*, *guilty*, *scared*, *mad*, and *surprised*. For this category, we relied on the theory of

Table 9.1 Three word categories patients use to describe emotional experiences

Word Code	Definition	Examples
Specific Feeling Words	Describe one specific, internal emotional experience	Angry, frustrated, bitter, sad, disgusted, anxious, happy, surprised, guilty
Vague Feeling Words	Refer to emotional experiences but do not refer to one feeling specifically	Bad, down, upset, emotional, distraught, overwhelmed, stressed
Physical Words	Describe *physical* experiences	Exhausted, tired, fatigued, calm, strong, achy, woozy, wobbly, dizzy, stiff

basic emotions, which asserts that certain feelings are identified universally by people from different cultural backgrounds and have distinct physical manifestations, particularly on the face (Ekman, 1992; Ekman and Friesen, 1971). While we did not limit specific feeling words to lists of basic emotions from the literature, we used the criterion that all the members of the research team had to be assured that they knew exactly what single feeling was being referenced to include the word as a specific feeling word. For instance, if reviewers found a respondent used the word *worried*, as long as everyone was satisfied that this word referred to a single emotional state (e.g., fear), then it was counted as a specific feeling word. What follows is an example from our data that was coded as a specific feeling word:

R: I got so *nervous*. [italics added]

Vague feeling words

In contrast, vague feeling words were words that clearly referred to some feeling state but did not clearly communicate one feeling state. For instance, when the respondent referred to feeling "pretty bad," reviewers could not tell whether bad was referring to any number of negative emotions, such as feeling sad, guilty, angry, or disgusted. Other examples of vague feeling words included feeling *down*, *upset*, *depressed*, or *stressed*.

Making a distinction between specific and vague feeling words was often challenging. Repeatedly during the development of the technique, reviewers made assumptions about the specific feeling state to which respondents were referring. For instance, some assumed that the word *depressed* automatically referred to feeling sad or that *stressed* always referred to anxiety. However, context often revealed that respondents used the word *depressed* paired with specific feelings of anger or fear and that *stressed* may similar refer to several feeling states (Yarns et al., 2018). It was therefore unknown whether *depressed* meant to convey sadness in addition to these other feelings, or whether it was a modification and elaboration of these other feelings that were specifically identified. This lack of clarity was exactly what characterized the vague feeling word category and distinguished it from the specific feeling word category. Here is another example from our data that was coded as a vague feeling word:

R: I feel *okay*. [italics added]

Physical words

Physical words were defined as words used to describe bodily internal – rather than emotional – experiences. Examples of physical words included *exhausted*, *tired*, *fatigued*, *nausea*, and *pain*. Some challenges also arose with classifying words that could refer either to emotional or physical experiences. Context was often helpful in making these distinctions. For instance, if a respondent said, "My arm *hurt*", then the word *hurt* was counted as a physical word. If a respondent said, "My feelings were *hurt*", then *hurt* was counted as a feeling word referring to emotional pain. We did not code medical diagnoses (e.g., *atrial fibrillation*), since these were not clear, explicit descriptions of a subjective, internal experience the respondent was having. Nor did we code phrases that did not include a single word that referred to a physical symptom. For instance, in the phrase "my heart beat faster", we did not include *heart*, *beat*, or *faster* as physical words, because we wanted to focus on single words that described a physical experience. Here is an example of what was coded as a physical word:

R: I have some, like, *dizziness*. [italics added]

Although PIC interviews were focused on understanding respondents' emotional experiences, we found numerous examples of physical words throughout every interview.

Reflections on using patterns of verbal expression of feelings in clinical practice

Overall, the approach of coding these three categories of words was viewed positively by both community and academic members of the research team. Team members described that after learning the word categories, they could hardly listen to their family or friends without noticing the words they use to describe their experience. One team member even commented that she believed learning the feeling word categories helped her own "emotional awareness". In addition, interrater reliability testing on 20% of our data resulted in kappa statistics between 0.94 and 1.0 for all three categories, indicating high interrater reliability.

We believe that learning and listening for patterns in the three categories of words that patients use to describe their emotional experience – specific feeling words, vague feeling words, and physical words – has several potential advantages for mental health professionals. Today, most mental health professionals are trained to listen to patients for content in order to make *DSM-5* diagnoses, rather than listening for subtle emotional information such as patterns of speech. However, as demonstrated, patients often have difficulty relaying the relevant content to their mental health provider. While it is true that our approach identifies certain types of content – three categories of words – the point for the clinician is to listen for patterns in the ways that patients describe their emotional experiences.

When speaking to patients, learning to listen for patterns in patients' descriptions of their emotional experiences using the three categories of words in the context of a discussion of feelings can augment self-report checklists, standard diagnostic interviews, and observing important nonverbal communication about feelings. To implement this type of listening, first a discussion of feelings must be opened. We encourage mental health professionals to ask frequently and repeatedly how the patient is feeling. We have found that mental health patients often present to their appointments describing some stressful event: a recent argument with a spouse, a stressful experience driving, or even disagreements with the clinic's front desk staff! If the patient comes into the mental health clinic visit reporting a recent stressful event, that can be the perfect opportunity to ask the patient about their feelings. Then, over time, the mental health professional can learn to recognise patterns in the patients' use of language to describe their feelings:

- Does the patient talk about feelings using specific feeling words?
- Are their responses vague?
- Despite repeated prompting for feelings, does the patient talk about physical experiences instead?
- Do they fail to answer the questions entirely?

Although further research is necessary, in our practice we have noted that different patterns in patients' verbal expression of feelings produces important diagnostic and prognostic information. We describe some of those observations in the paragraphs that follow. In addition, we have discovered that certain interviewing strategies can help patients develop new and more communicative ways of expressing their feelings.

The benefits of specific feeling words

We believe that specific feeling words provide mental health professionals with more actionable information than vague feeling words or physical words, and that mental health professionals should work to try to elicit specific feelings from patients. First, eliciting specific feeling words from patients can empower clinicians to provide more precise strategies to help patients cope with specific feelings they are experiencing. For example, if patients feel comfortable voicing anger and frustration, then mental health professionals can help patients set boundaries or assert themselves in a constructive way. If patients express guilt, then mental health professionals can help them figure out how to repair the bond or relationship the patients' actions may have put at risk.

Second, eliciting specific feeling words can augment other strategies, such as traditional clinical interviews and self-report checklists, to help mental health professionals make accurate diagnoses. For instance, a substantial literature focuses on the clinical imperative to distinguish between normal grief and clinical depression (Friedman, 2012). After the loss of a loved one, it is natural for patients to feel several feelings: especially sadness, but sometimes also guilt and anger at the deceased are part of a normal grieving process. While grief is expected to resolve on its own, that is not always the case (Maciejewski et al., 2007). If the mental health professional can elicit the specific feelings the grieving patient is experiencing, they can be supported and helped to work through these feelings. Normal grieving may then be diagnosed and facilitated rather than diagnosed as a clinical entity and prescribed medication.

What to do with vague feeling words

Patients who tend to describe their emotional experience primarily with vague feeling words often provide mental health professionals with less actionable information. Patients who come into clinic reporting they are feeling "bad" or "upset" are not conveying a clear picture of what the mental health professional can do to help them. In our clinical experience, patients who primarily use vague words to describe often have a history of difficult interactions with mental health professionals and may also report a pattern of receiving little help. For patients who rely on vague feeling words, it may be useful to repeat questions about feelings often and encourage them to be specific.

In cases where vague feelings are used repeatedly despite gentle encouragement to be specific, we recommend a three-step process, originally described by Davanloo (Davanloo, 1990). First, *point out* that the patient is using a vague word to describe their emotional experience. Clinicians may simply state, "When you say you are feeling 'bad', that is vague". Second, describe the *function* of the vagueness: "Staying vague is a way you keep us from understanding your feelings". And third, identify the *cost* of continuing to be vague: "If we don't understand specifically what you are feeling, then it makes it impossible for us to figure out the kind of specific help you need". If a patient continues to use vague words, this may hold important prognostic information about whether the patient is able to communicate their distress and obtain the help they need. For instance, vague speech has been associated with difficult-to-treat conditions, including some personality disorders (Pfohl, 1991).

Physical words and emotional experience

Finally, if a patient primarily communicates about emotional experience using physical words, this can also provide important diagnostic and prognostic information. However, a patient providing information about physical symptoms may not provide actionable information for the mental health professional. After all, most mental health professionals do not provide diagnosis and treatment of physical health conditions.

The reader may be unclear about why we report physical words as a category of emotional experience. However, our data set revealed numerous examples of interviewers clearly asking for emotional experience and instead getting descriptions of physical experience. For years, mental health professionals and researchers have noted an overlap of emotional and physical experience. For instance, in *Studies on Hysteria*, Breuer and Freud wrote that patients such as the famed Anna O. could be cured of disabling physical symptoms by recalling the feelings that accompanied each instance of the symptom all the way back to the first instance (Freud et al., 1971). While Breuer and Freud's cases have come under increased scrutiny in recent decades, more recent theory and empirical research focus on how physical sensations in the body are important components of emotional experience (Davanloo, 2001; Kleinman, 1982; MacCormack and Lindquist, 2017; Scherer, 2005). And neuroimaging data now highlight the overlap in brain circuitry involved in physical and emotional experiences such as physical and emotional pain and hunger (Eisenberger and Lieberman, 2004; MacCormack and Lindquist, 2019).

Finally, research suggests that some physical symptoms – especially certain types of chronic pain – may be understood as emotional experiences, which are generated due to psychological conflict rather than injury in peripheral tissues (Lumley et al., 2011). The term *central sensitivity syndromes* refers to physical health conditions that are thought to be mostly or entirely due to activity in the central nervous system (Yunus, 2007). Further research is necessary to determine whether speech patterns can be used to establish the presence of central sensitivity syndromes. Yet, clearly the literature asserts considerable overlap between emotional symptoms and physical symptoms.

The key to assessing physical words using our criteria is that the clinician should make sure it is done in the context of a conversation about feelings. If mental health professionals ask about specific feelings and receive statements on physical symptoms instead, then this understanding can inform how the clinician approaches the patient over many visits, such as asking about physical pain in ways that also incorporate space for emotional experience. For instance, the mental health clinician can provide psychoeducation about the effects of feelings on physical symptoms and the importance of discussing emotional as well as physical experiences. As with vague feeling words, the mental health professional may also use specific techniques such as repeating a question and clarifying the cost of focusing on physical symptoms to the exclusion of feelings during a mental health visit.

However, mental health professionals should be sensitive to the patient's perspective about the origins of their physical symptoms. In our experience, patients who use physical words to discuss emotional experiences usually do not initially understand that they are using physical words to describe emotional distress and may feel misunderstood if the clinician is too heavy-handed in helping them make a distinction between their physical and emotional experiences. Also, at times patients do discuss their physical

---

Box 9.1   Practical tips

Practical tips for improving communication

- Ask about feelings often.
- Listen for whether patients tend to use *specific feeling words, vague feeling words*, or *physical words*.
- Help patients cope with the specific feelings they are experiencing.
- Ask for specificity if patients tend to use vague feeling words.
- Give space to incorporate emotional experience in patients who tend to only discuss their physical experiences.

---

health conditions with mental health professionals to receive emotional support. In our experience, this is perfectly appropriate and does not imply overlap between physical and mental health symptoms. If a clinician attempts to label physical words as emotional experiences prior to significant exploration with the patient and without explicitly setting up the boundaries of the conversation as a discussion of feelings, then patients can feel hurt and a misalliance can develop.

However, occasionally patients are receptive to a referral for psychotherapy to understand the relationship between their physical and emotional experiences. In these cases, empirical research, including our own, suggests that patients can receive benefits on some physical symptoms, especially chronic pain (Lumley and Schubiner, 2019). Improving emotional awareness, experience, and healthy expression of adaptive emotions through written emotional disclosure or psychotherapy has proven beneficial for several patient populations with mind-body syndromes, including patients with irritable bowel syndrome (Thakur et al., 2017) and chronic pain (Burger et al., 2016; Graham et al., 2008; Hsu et al., 2010; Lumley et al., 2017; Pepe et al., 2014). One of us (B.C.Y.) recently completed a preliminary clinical trial comparing emotional awareness and expression therapy (EAET) and cognitive behavioural therapy (CBT) for older veterans with chronic musculoskeletal pain and found significant advantages of EAET over CBT in this population (Najafian Jazi et al., 2019). To summarise, therefore, we offer some practical tips in Box 9.1.

Conclusions

In summary, patients often have complex and even baffling responses to seemingly simple questions about their feelings. Using a theoretical framework derived from both conceptual and empirical research on emotions, we developed a technique to aide in understanding complex communications about feelings and assessing patterns in the way patients describe their emotional experiences. The result was three qualitatively different categories of words: specific feeling words, vague feeling words, and physical words. Clinicians can notice which categories individual patients tend to use to describe their feelings and make specific interventions in each case. For specific feeling words, which we believe provide the best information for mental health professionals, clinicians can help patients work through the specific feelings that patients are experiencing. For instance, if a patient is sad, the clinician can help the patient grieve. If a patient uses mostly vague words to describe their feeling, clinicians can help the patient to be more specific and understand how specificity and detail are most likely to get them the help they need. If patient tends to use more physical words to describe their emotional experience, the mental health professional can allow space and encouragement for the patient to discuss their emotional experiences as well. It is our hope that this kind of "listening for experiencing" can augment other strategies mental health professionals use to assess their patients' feelings, such as the clinical interview and self-report checklists.

Required Disclaimer: "These contents do not represent the views of the U.S. Department of Veterans Affairs or the United States Government."

Sources of Support: This work was supported by a grant from the U.S. Department of Veterans Affairs (grant number CX001884).

References

American Psychiatric Association, 2013. *Diagnostic and statistical manual of mental disorders (DSM-5®)*. American Psychiatric Association, Arlington, VA.

Bagby, R.M., Parker, J.D., Taylor, G.J., 1994. The twenty-item Toronto Alexithymia Scale-I: Item selection and cross-validation of the factor structure. *J. Psychosom. Res.* 38 (1), 23–32.

Barrett, J.E., Barrett, J.A., Oxman, T.E., Gerber, P.D., 1988. The prevalence of psychiatric disorders in a primary care practice. *Arch. Gen. Psychiatry* 45 (12), 1100–1106.

Bhatia, M., Rodriguez, M.G., Fowler, D.M., Godin, J.E., Drapeau, M., McCullough, L., 2009. Desensitization of conflicted feelings: Using the ATOS to measure early change in a single-case affect phobia therapy treatment. *Archives of Psychiatry & Psychotherapy* 11 (1), 31–38.

Borowsky, S.J., Rubenstein, L.V., Meredith, L.S., Camp, P., Jackson-Triche, M., Wells, K.B., 2000. Who Is at Risk of Nondetection of Mental Health Problems in Primary Care? *Journal of General Internal Medicine* 15 (6), 381–388. doi:10.1046/j.1525-1497.2000.12088.x.

Briggs, J.L., 1970. *Never in Anger: Portrait of an Eskimo Family,* vol. 12. Harvard University Press, Cambridge, MA.

Bromley, E., Kennedy, D.P., Miranda, J., Sherbourne, C.D., Wells, K.B., 2016. The fracture of relational space in depression: Predicaments in primary care help seeking. *Current Anthropology* 57 (5), 610–631. doi:10.1086/688506.

Burger, A.J., Lumley, M.A., Carty, J.N., Latsch, D.V., Thakur, E.R., Hyde-Nolan,

M.E., Schubiner, H., 2016. The effects of a novel psychological attribution and emotional awareness and expression therapy for chronic musculoskeletal pain: A preliminary, uncontrolled trial. *Journal of Psychosomatic Research* 81, 1–8.

Capps, L., Ochs, E., 1995. *Constructing Panic*. Harvard University Press, Cambridge, MA.

Cowie, R., Douglas-Cowie, E., Tsapatsoulis, N., Votsis, G., Kollias, S., Fellenz, W., Taylor, J.G., 2001. Emotion recognition in human-computer interaction. *IEEE Signal Processing Magazine* 18 (1), 32–80.

Davanloo, H., 1990. *Unlocking the Unconscious: Selected Papers of Habib Davanloo*. Wiley, New York.

Davanloo, H., 2001. Intensive short-term dynamic psychotherapy: extended major direct access to the unconscious. *European Psychotherapy* 2 (2), 25–70.

DeSteno, D., Gross, J.J., Kubzansky, L., 2013. Affective science and health: The importance of emotion and emotion regulation. *Health Psychology* 32 (5), 474–486.

Eisenberger, N.I., Lieberman, M.D., 2004. Why rejection hurts: A common neural alarm system for physical and social pain. *Trends in Cognitive Sciences* 8 (7), 294–300.

Ekman, P., 1992. An argument for basic emotions. *Cognition & Emotion* 6 (3–4), 169–200.

Ekman, P., Friesen, W.V., 1971. Constants across cultures in the face and emotion. *Journal of Personality and Social Psychology* 17 (2), 124–129. 10.1037/h0030377.

Else-Quest, N.M., Higgins, A., Allison, C., Morton, L.C., 2012. Gender differences in self conscious emotional experience: A meta-analysis. *Psychological Bulletin 138* (5), 947–981.

Fledderus, M., Bohlmeijer, E.T., Pieterse, M.E., 2010. Does experiential avoidance mediate the effects of maladaptive coping styles on psychopathology and mental health? *Behavior Modification* 34 (6), 503–519.

Freud, A., 1966. *The Ego and the Mechanisms of Defense* (C. Baines, Trans.). Hogarth, London, UK (original work published 1936).

Freud, S., 1936. *Inhibitions, Anxiety, and Symptoms*. (A. Strachey, Trans.). Longmans, Green, Toronto (original work published 1926).

Freud, S., Breuer, J., Strachey, J., Freud, A., 1971. *Studies on Hysteria* (A. Strachey, Trans.). Longmans, Green, Toronto (original work published 1895).

Frewen, P.A., Dozois, D.J., Neufeld, R.W., Lanius, R.A., 2008. Meta-analysis of alexithymia in posttraumatic stress disorder. *J Trauma Stress* 21 (2), 243–246. doi:10.1002/jts.20320.

Friedman, R.A., 2012. Grief, depression, and the DSM-5. *N Engl J Med* 366 (*20*), 1855–1857.

Graham, J.E., Lobel, M., Glass, P., Lokshina, I., 2008. Effects of written anger expression in chronic pain patients: Making meaning from pain. *J Behav Med* 31 (3), 201–212.

Hayes, S.C., Strosahl, K.D., Wilson, K.G., 1999. *Acceptance and Commitment Therapy: An Experiential Approach to Behavior Change*. Guilford Press, New York.

Hayes, S.C., Wilson, K.G., Gifford, E.V., Follette, V.M., Strosahl, K., 1996. Experiential avoidance and behavioral disorders: A functional dimensional approach to diagnosis and treatment. *Journal of Consulting and Clinical Psychology* 64 (6), 1152.

Hsu, M.C., Schubiner, H., Lumley, M.A., Stracks, J.S., Clauw, D.J., Williams, D.A., 2010. Sustained pain reduction through affective self-awareness in fibromyalgia: A randomized controlled trial. *Journal of General Internal Medicine* 25 (10), 1064–1070.

King, L.A., Emmons, R.A., 1990. Conflict over emotional expression: Psychological and physical correlates. *J. Pers. Soc. Psychol.* 58 (5), 864–877.

Kirmayer, L.J., 1989. Cultural variations in the response to psychiatric disorders and emotional distress. *Soc. Sci. Med.* 29 (3), 327–339. doi:10.1016/0277-9536(89)90281-5.

Kleinman, A., 1982. Neurasthenia and depression: A study of somatization and culture in China. *Culture, Medicine and Psychiatry* 6 (2), 117–190.

Kojima, M., 2012. Alexithymia as a prognostic risk factor for health problems: A brief review of epidemiological studies. *BioPsychoSocial Medicine* 6 (1), 21.

Kroenke, K., Spitzer, R.L., Williams, J.B., 2001. The PHQ-9: Validity of a brief depression severity measure. *J. Gen. Intern. Med.* 16 (9), 606–613.

Kroenke, K., Spitzer, R.L., Williams, J.B., 2003. The Patient Health Questionnaire-2: Validity of a two-item depression screener. *Medical Care* 41 (11), 1284–1292.

Lane, R.D., Weihs, K.L., Herring, A., Hishaw, A., Smith, R., 2015. Affective agnosia: Expansion of the alexithymia construct and a new opportunity to integrate and extend Freud's legacy. *Neurosci. Biobehav. Rev.* 55, 594–611. doi:10.1016/j.neubiorev.2015.06.007.

Lumley, M.A., Cohen, J.L., Borszcz, G.S., Cano, A., Radcliffe, A.M., Porter, L.S., Keefe, F.J., 2011. Pain and emotion: A biopsychosocial review of recent research. *Journal of Clinical Psychology* 67 (9), 942–968.

Lumley, M.A., Schubiner, H., 2019. Psychological therapy for centralized pain: An integrative assessment and treatment model. *Psychosomatic Medicine* 81 (2), 114–124.

Lumley, M.A., Schubiner, H., Lockhart, N.A., Kidwell, K.M., Harte, S.E., Clauw, D.J., Williams, D.A., 2017. Emotional awareness and expression therapy, cognitive behavioral therapy, and education for fibromyalgia: A cluster-randomized controlled trial. *Pain* 158 (12), 2354–2363.

MacCormack, J.K., Lindquist, K.A., 2017. Bodily contributions to emotion: Schachter's legacy for a psychological constructionist view on emotion. *Emotion Review* 9 (1), 36–45.

MacCormack, J.K., Lindquist, K.A., 2019. Feeling hangry? When hunger is conceptualized as emotion. *Emotion* 19 (2), 301–319.

McCullough, L., 2003. *Treating Affect Phobia: A Manual for Short-Term Dynamic Psychotherapy*. Guilford Press, New York.

Maciejewski, P.K., Zhang, B., Block, S.D., Prigerson, H.G., 2007. An empirical examination of the stage theory of grief. *JAMA* 297 (7), 716–723.

Moussavi, S., Chatterji, S., Verdes, E., Tandon, A., Patel, V., Ustun, B., 2007. Depression, chronic diseases, and decrements in health: Results from the World Health Surveys. *Lancet* 370 (9590), 851–858. doi:10.1016/s0140-6736(07)61415-9.

Najafian Jazi, A., Sultzer, D.L., Lumley, M.A., Osato, S., Yarns, B.C., 2019. Emotional awareness and expression therapy (EAET) or cognitive behavior therapy (CBT) for the treatment of chronic musculoskeletal pain in older veterans: A pilot randomized clinical trial. *Am. J. Geriatr. Psychiatry* 27 (3), S153–S154.

Panksepp, J., 1998. *Affective Neuroscience: The Foundations of Human and Animal Emotions.* Oxford University Press, Oxford.

Pepe, L., Milani, R., Di Trani, M., Di Folco, G., Lanna, V., Solano, L., 2014. A more global approach to musculoskeletal pain: Expressive writing as an effective adjunct to physiotherapy. *Psychology, Health & Medicine* 19 (6), 687–697.

Pfohl, B., 1991. Histrionic personality disorder: A review of available data and recommendations for DSM-IV. *Journal of Personality Disorders* 5 (2), 150–166.

Rubenstein, L.V., Jackson-Triche, M., Unutzer, J., Miranda, J., Minnium, K., Pearson, M.L., Wells, K.B., 1999. Evidence-based care for depression in managed primary care practices. *Health Affairs* 18 (5), 89–105.

Scherer, K.R., 2005. What are emotions? And how can they be measured? *Social Science Information* 44 (4), 695–729.

Schoenbaum, M., Unützer, J., Sherbourne, C., Duan, N., Rubenstein, L.V., Miranda, J., Wells, K., 2001. Cost-effectiveness of practice-initiated quality improvement for depression: Results of a randomized controlled trial. *JAMA* 286 (11), 1325–1330.

Shapiro, J., 2011. Perspective: Does medical education promote professional alexithymia? A call for attending to the emotions of patients and self in medical training. *Academic Medicine* 86 (3), 326–332.

Sherbourne, C.D., Wells, K.B., Duan, N., Miranda, J., Unützer, J., Jaycox, L., Rubenstein, L.V., 2001. Long-term effectiveness of disseminating quality improvement for depression in primary care. *Archives of General Psychiatry* 58 (7), 696–703.

Sifneos, P.E., Apfel-Savitz, R., Frankel, F.H., 1977. The phenomenon of "alexithymia". Observations in neurotic and psychosomatic patients. *Psychother Psychosom* 28 (1–4), 47–57.

Spitzer, R.L., Kroenke, K., Williams, J.B., Löwe, B., 2006. A brief measure for assessing generalized anxiety disorder: The GAD-7. *Archives of Internal Medicine* 166 (10), 1092–1097.

Thakur, E., Holmes, H., Lockhart, N., Carty, J., Ziadni, M., Doherty, H., Lumley, M., 2017. Emotional awareness and expression training improves irritable bowel syndrome: A randomized controlled trial. *Neurogastroenterol. Motil.* 29 (12). doi:10.1111/nmo.13143.

Vaillant, L.M., 1997. *Changing Character: Short-Term Anxiety-Regulating Psychotherapy for Restructuring Defenses, Affects, and Attachment.* Basic Books, New York.

Wells, K., Sherbourne, C., Schoenbaum, M., Ettner, S., Duan, N., Miranda, J., Rubenstein, L., 2004. 5-year impact of quality improvement for depression: Results of a group-level randomized controlled trial. *Archives of General Psychiatry* 61 (4), 378–386.

Wells, K.B., 1999. The design of Partners in Care: evaluating the cost-effectiveness of improving care for depression in primary care. *Soc. Psychiatry Psychiatr. Epidemiol.* 34 (1), 20–29.

Wells, K.B., Sherbourne, C., Schoenbaum, M., Duan, N., Meredith, L., Unützer, J., Rubenstein, L.V., 2000. Impact of disseminating quality improvement programs for depression in managed primary care: a randomized controlled trial. *JAMA 283* (2), 212–220.

Williams, K.E., Chambless, D.L., Ahrens, A., 1997. Are emotions frightening? An extension of the fear of fear construct. *Behav. Res. Ther.* 35 (3), 239–248.

Wrenn, K.C., Mostofsky, E., Tofler, G.H., Muller, J.E., Mittleman, M.A., 2013. Anxiety, anger, and mortality risk among survivors of myocardial infarction. *Am. J. Med.* 126 (12), 1107–1113. doi:10.1016/j.amjmed.2013.07.022.

Yarns, B.C., Wells, K.B., Fan, D., Mtume, N., Bromley, E., 2018. The physical and the emotional: Case report, mixed-methods development, and discussion. *Psychodynamic Psychiatry* 46 (4), 553–578.

Yunus, M.B., 2007. Fibromyalgia and overlapping disorders: The unifying concept of central sensitivity syndromes. *Semin. Arthritis Rheum.* 36 (6), 339–356. doi:10.1016/j.semarthrit.2006.12.009.

Chapter 10

Communication in mental health nursing

The power of the words we choose

Mary Farrelly

Introduction

Nursing can be understood as a "textually mediated reality" (Cheek 1993, Cheek and Rudge, 1994a, p. 15) in which our understandings of the realities of practice are constituted by the language we use and which in turn constitute the language we use. Examination of and reflection on the "taken for granted" realities implicit in our communication is an important part of developing helpful communication. This chapter will consider the issues of communication in mental health nursing through an exploration of the use of language. Mental health nurses are arguably the professional occupational group who are engaged in the most sustained communication with people who experience mental health problems and their families and supporters across all settings and over the full 24-hour, 7-day period. As such, we also have a pivotal role in communicating with other professionals and staff about service users. In our everyday lives and in wider society we are frequently viewed as having authority on issues of mental health. Mental health nurses are frequently required to provide explanations for service users, families, and others about the nature of mental distress (Crowe, 2000) and how we do that, and what discourses we draw on, has consequences for how understandings of mental health are constituted, with important effects for those affected. In short, the language we use about mental health matters.

Drawing on research that considers the constitutive nature of language, this chapter considers research that has examined the way in which language makes meaning of mental health issues and how language, used by mental health nurses and other professionals in communication with service users, their families, and the public has important consequences. Particular attention will be paid to how the use of psychiatrically oriented language and pessimistic talk can produce particular versions of reality that are unhelpful, contesting the rhetoric of recovery. Mental health nursing verbal and written communication will be considered from a variety of perspectives; communication with service users and families, with other workers and in wider public fora. Recommendations for practice and clinical scenarios will be provided to illustrate real-life examples, of issues such as discussing diagnosis, conveying optimism and hope, and care planning.

Language and mental health

The consideration and analysis of discourse is important in gaining an understanding of meaning, knowledge, and power in relation to mental health problems. For much of the general public their primary access to information about mental health is through media sources. Media is recognized as a significant social site where meaning is constructed, forming societal understandings of what constitutes "mental health problems" and constituting notions of causation, appropriate responses, and treatments. A major area of research on language and mental health has been concerned with media representation. The manner in which mental health problems are represented and understood has important consequences for those who experience them (and others) but the issue of how meaning about mental health is made has wider implications beyond individual attitudes; it has potential to impact on personal identity, self-esteem, help seeking behaviour, and stigmatization. Another major area for investigation has been mental health nurses' communication with services users, their relatives and supporters, and other nurses and members of the multidisciplinary team formally at meetings and handovers and informally in conversations and through documentation in notes and reports.

Media research

Media coverage of mental health problems is widespread in newsprint, television, radio, and online (Francis et al., 2004; Diefenbach, 1997; Philo, Henderson, and McCracken, 2010; Wahl and Roth, 1982). A considerable body of research indicates that mental health problems are portrayed in a negative manner in mass media, both in news and entertainment, print and broadcast. Studies demonstrate an association of mental health problems with violence and aggression, depiction of negative stereotypical images, comic representation, use of pejorative or negative colloquial terms to convey mental health problems (McGinty et al., 2014; Philo et al., 2010; Bilić and Georgaca, 2007; Coverdale, Nairn, and Claasen, 2002; Nairn, Coverdale, and Claasen, 2001; Wilson et al., 1999a,b; Allen and Nairn, 1997) and conflation with risk, criminality, violence, lack of personal agency and biomedical understandings by media (Hazelton, 1997). Given the ubiquity of mental health problems in media sources, it is fair to conclude that the general public have a large exposure related to mental health that is likely to influence their understanding of mental health problems, the formation of attitudes and influence their behaviour both in relation to their own mental health and to people who experience mental ill-health. Popular media is an important source of knowledge for the public about "mental illness" (Dietrich et al., 2006; Angermeyer et al., 2005; Penn, Chamberlin, and Mueser, 2003; Granello, Pauley, and Carmichael, 1999; Thornton and Wahl, 1996; Daniel Yanklovich Group Inc., 1990). Some studies suggest that the more television an individual watches the more likely they are to express opinions and hold views similar to those represented on the television (Stout, Villegas, and Jennings, 2004; Gerbner et al., 1986) and that "negative" media coverage contributes to negative attitudes towards people with mental health problems (Morgan and Jorm, 2009; Thornton and Wahl, 1996). This understanding has formed the basis of anti-stigma initiatives and guidelines on reporting that emphasise positive stereotypes and the use of "appropriate" language. Such research offers insight into the formation of knowledge and the operation of power in making meaning about mental health. Many of these guidelines and campaigns promote medicalised definitions by making comparisons with physical illness and foregrounding professional knowledge.

My study of media representation in Irish newspapers considered the ways in which mental health problems were discursively constructed involved an analysis of 123 news items with mental health content to consider the way meaning was made about mental health problems (Farrelly, 2015). Mental health problems were constructed by enlisting a range of discursive categories. For example, my research highlighted that mental health problems were constructed as being hidden due to stigma and elusiveness of definition and this "hiddenness" was defined by not "coming to the attention of the authorities". Hiddenness was considered problematic due to a risk of danger to the person and as a barrier to receiving help. The dominant means of achieving visibility, "obtaining a diagnosis", foregrounds psychiatric definition of mental distress obscuring other possible meanings or forms of expressions.

To give a specific example this extract from an article on obsessive compulsive disorder (OCD) states:

> American research indicates that people with OCD see three to four doctors and spend more than 9 years seeking treatment before they receive a correct diagnosis. OCD is difficult to diagnose and people suffering from the disorder are often secretive about their symptoms or lack insight into their illness. It's even difficult to describe the condition. Other studies have found that it takes an average of 17 years for people to obtain appropriate treatment from the time OCD begins. OCD has been misdiagnosed as depression, bipolar disorder, ADHD, autism and schizophrenia. Getting proper diagnosis and appropriate treatment can take even longer in Ireland, according to (psychologist and adviser to OCD organisation). (Cycle of obsessive thoughts. Irish Times. Healthplus Supplement, 13 January, 2009, p. 7)

The reasons for OCD not being recognized are given as:

1.   It is difficult to diagnose correctly.
2.   Many doctors may not recognize it.
3.   It is difficult to describe.
4.   People keep it a secret.
5.   People who have it do not understand that they have it.

The explanations provided for the invisibility of OCD function to support the existence of an objective reality, a diagnosis called OCD, a "proper diagnosis". Increased awareness was the normative response to the problem of hiddenness. Several ways of increasing the visibility of mental health problems were privileged. The imperative to be diagnosed is privileged, with warnings of the difficulties in getting a diagnosis and advice to self-diagnose. Diagnosis is only problematized in so much as it is difficult to get it right, the blame lies with the "condition" or the "practitioner", there is no questioning of the ideological or scientific basis for the diagnostic framework. Raising awareness was to be achieved by providing more information about "it", alerting others to watch out for 'it', and encouraging people who experience 'it' to talk about 'it'. This logic underpins mental health policy and mental health promotion campaigns that promote greater awareness and encourage people to be open and frank about their mental health problems with the aims of alleviating stigma and encouraging people to seek help. While this may well be helpful for people who experience mental distress, in terms of de-stigmatization, the mechanisms legitimized for producing such awareness are not neutral. In other words, the methods we employ for de-stigmatization lead to categorization. The normative means of naming mental distress and the mechanisms for measuring it and bringing into public discourse construct 'it' as "mental illness", a health problem of the individual, the concern of psychiatry. Another way is by increasing the likelihood of it being defined by making diagnostic mechanisms more amenable and available and by suggesting that this is the route to care. By legitimizing diagnostic systems for identifying mental health problems in this way, biomedical, psychiatric meanings of mental health problems are normalized and other ways of giving expression to mental distress, as "problems of living" (Tszaz, 1974) for example, are obscured or disallowed. This reinforces the existence of a particular type of mental distress, an entity called "mental illness" or "mental disorder" bringing it into the domain of medicine. The preferencing of an approach that leads to diagnosis results in other means of understanding and helping what the person is experiencing being shut down.

Categories of crises, risk, and danger constructed mental health problems in newspapers as increasing and as dangerous and devastating to the person in terms of their functioning, agency and selfhood, impacting others in a negative way. This produces an understanding of people with mental health problems as having little or no control and is likely to engender fear, discomfort towards people with mental health problems and impact on their own self-esteem and self-worth. It potentially diminishes the person with a mental health problem by portraying them in a negative light and locates the imperative for action with outside agency. It produces an "inept" person incapable of taking responsibility and obscures possibilities of recovery and potentially deprives people who experience mental health problems of agency in managing their own lives and taking responsibility for their recovery. This further reinforces societal stigma in relation to mental health problems and produces a need for the external government of mental health and the individual. It individualizes societal problems, constituting feelings such as sadness, dissatisfaction, disappointment, regret, and unhappiness that are frequently a result of difficulties encountered with the way the world is organized and associated with poverty, unemployment, social disadvantage, homelessness, and marginalization, as pathological states, "mental health problems" or "mental illness". My study found, where recovery was deemed possible dominant professional discourses that emphasized adherence to treatment, medication, and acceptance of biomedical diagnosis were prevalent. The dominant normative response to mental health problems was engagement with mental health services which were the "taken for granted" best response to mental health problems. Such constructions operate to produce an understanding of mental health problems and mental distress as being an individual, biomedically defined phenomenon, beyond the control of the individual, dangerous and devastating to the person, others, and society, constructing mental health problems as outside the locus and control of people who experience them, producing a need for the government of mental health. Psychiatric knowledge was privileged and uncontested as the legitimate means of both making mental distress visible and as a means of response with important implications for people experiencing mental health problems, their supporters, and for society as a whole in making meaning about mental distress and for the forms of help that can be made available to them. Critical discourses that challenge the legitimacy of biological explanations and psychiatry were largely absent.

Over the past 20 years, Internet and social media have become major sites of social interaction. Research into mental health and Internet and social media has been concerned mainly with issues such as the effects of social media use on the mental health of users, representations of various mental health difficulties such as depression, eating disorders and borderline personality disorder, and the potential of online media to contribute to mental health education and treatments. For example, links between use of social networks such as Facebook and Twitter and low self-esteem have been identified, notwithstanding difficulties identifying cause and effect (Pantnic, 2014). Like research on print and televisual media research, the dominance of professionalized discourses has been identified in considerations of social media and representations of mental health problems. Dyson and Gorvin (2017) identified from a sample of "Tweets" by people who identified as having "Borderline Personality Disorder" that participants constructed themselves with recourse to a biomedical repertoire by identifying as "victims of a disorder". This, and the "intrinsic nature" of the "disorder", operated to exonerate them from responsibility for behaviour and engagement with treatment, creating a pessimistic view of the possibility for change. Online platforms have provided opportunities for various interest groups to "meet" and share experiences, advice, and support. Participation in Facebook groups such as Mad Pride International, Intervoice, Mad in America, and online sites which are focussed on particular mental health problems, however, require identification with particular discursive constructions. Adopting certain terms to refer to personal experience and distress positions the experience and potential responses. Sites which are titled "Voice Hearing" or "Survivorship" indicate alignment with critical perspectives on mental health and participating in a social media group related to depression, anorexia, or borderline personality disorder requires the person to identify with the relevant diagnostic category (Giles and Newbold, 2011). Charland (2004) suggests that psychiatric labels are maintained by consumers in such fora even after they have been abolished by the medical establishment and that consumer autonomy and the Internet are now powerful new forces in the manufacture of madness (p. 335).

Nursing and professional communication

The way in which mental health nurses and other professionals communicate with and about service users is another important area for consideration. Communication among staff happens formally in team meetings, at handovers and case conferences (see Dobbinson, this volume and Drewett, this volume, for discussion of inpatient settings) and informally in conversations, and in written forms in reports, care plans, and referral letters, for example. It can have direct effects on service-users' well-being and behaviour. Staff communication with clients has been shown to impact on levels of aggression and violence. A study of staff-patient interaction in an Irish adult mental health service suggested that some critical incidents arise from the staff's lack of consistent engagement with patients (Moore, 2017). A large programme of research in UK acute psychiatric wards (Safewards Project) investigated variation in episodes of conflict (absconding, aggression, rule breaking, medication refusal, self-harm, and suicide) and containment practices (seclusion, PRN and coerced medication, special observation, and manual restraint) and found that the nature and quality of staff communication and interaction with patients is an important contributing factor to the frequency of these adverse events (Bowers, 2014, Bowers et al., 2011).

A study of verbal communication of risk at handovers in an acute psychiatric unit highlighted the subjective and contingent nature of information communicated amongst staff (Millar and Sands, 2010). They revealed inconsistencies in reporting with ambiguous, superfluous terms; irrelevant information; and the nature and amount of information being communicated being inconsistent with information in patient records and varying depending on time of day, method of communication, nurses' familiarity with the patient, and type of handover. Communication was mainly verbal, leading to information being frequently re-produced with increasing inaccuracies depending on the number of times it had been reproduced. Another study of verbal communication between staff members about patients in a psychiatric day unit described episodes of communication where descriptions of patients' behaviours were summarized and reformulated in a professionalized language of psychopathology, "a tendency which rapidly foreclosed the possibility of generating alternative or conflicting interpretations from the original material" (Allen, 1981, p. 357). One such interaction is described:

Psychologist: "What was it her sister said? She can't keep her mind on anything ... a ... what was it? A butterfly?"
Senior registrar: "Yes, there's this terrible failure of concentration."
Nurse: "She'll be talking to you and suddenly she'll be on a quite different ... like the thing about the teeth."
Consultant: "Yes, that was quite glaring. I think you're quite right. There's this *underlying manic tendency*, one feels."

This brief extract demonstrates how a metaphor such as "like a butterfly" gets transformed into medicalised language leading to diagnostic categorisation, of "underlying manic tendency". The study also provided evidence of prognostic pessimism in the way staff spoke about patients, predicting relapse and poor outcomes. Allen concluded that much of the talk could be reduced to a single message: "patients are not like us" (p. 362).

Cheek and Rudge (1994a,b) considering case notes suggest that the "patient" is constructed by the operation of dominant discourses and personal knowledge and the voice of the patient is muted by "webs of documentation". They describe how patients are effectively "absent" in their notes as the professional voice is dominant and then further excluded from those notes by not being allowed access to them. Talking about the language that is used and how observations are shaped they say:

To illustrate the application of some of the issues raised, you might like to pause to consider language use in your own practice context. Often in the course of the day, you develop concerns about a particular patient's condition. At first these concerns may be no more than hunches, or in other words, subjective meanings. First of all, you may discuss your concerns with colleagues on the shift and try to put into words your suspicions about the patient. To do this you will be using established signs and language that act as representations of your previously unvoiced concerns. These interactions with others may still remain more in the realm of shared subjective concerns, but nurses are also expected to "report" these changes in patient status. At this stage, you are forced into particular practices – you write a report in the case notes. The basis for your report may well be the nursing process, with its diagnostic statements, or some other form of ordering your, as yet, unsubstantiated concerns. The language and the form of reporting you use will now be formed by the rules that govern such reporting. In the process, your concerns will be reported as changes in the biological parameters (scientific/medical language), objective statements of the patient's condition (medical/legal language), and "nursing diagnosis" and evaluations of interventions (nursing dogma). In this process, what was initially "a personal opinion" has come to be registered as objective fact. Nursing knowledge is converted into the language and meanings of medical/scientific discourse.

(Cheek and Rudge, 1994a, p. 17)

The use of classification systems, like DSM-5, nursing diagnoses, tools such as standardised care plans, while helpful from a management perspective in the organisation of care, require the use of standardised language. This makes possible what Foucault refers to as "technologies of normalization" (Irving et al., 2006, p. 152) rendering the individual human experience invisible, or visible only in so much as it is defined by particular knowledge, usually biomedical. Authoritarian, professionalized language defines the person in a particular way, thus limiting the possibilities for understanding the person and care (Cheek and Rudge, 1993). A psychiatric diagnosis legitimizes interventions as treatments which alter the course of a condition rather than just supressing symptoms and eradicates culpability for actions and exempts people from usual criminal justice system sanctions for example (Moncrieff, 2010) thereby diminishing personal responsibility and obscuring social processes as implicated in human distress.

Implications for mental health nursing practice

The previous section highlights the constitutive nature of language in constructing versions of reality revealing dominant discourses. Language is a disciplinary practice that mediates power and its consequences for those who are its subjects. Recognizing that all language is constitutive, the challenge is to choose to communicate and select ways of communicating that are helpful for services users and society in understanding and dealing with mental distress. A key element of helpful communication is the ability to reflect on the meaning our words convey. Mental health nurses need to be able to use language in their talk with and about the people the care for that acknowledges the uniqueness of the individual and enables them to flourish rather than language dominated by colloquial or technical terminology that pigeonholes them into a social or diagnostic category which diminishes their personhood. This applies to communication with patients and relatives, communication about patients with other staff, communication with the wider community. It applies to verbal communication in conversation, nursing interventions, handovers, team meetings, case conferences, and on media or in public fora, as well as in written communication in care plans, case notes, referral letters, and media content. Two particular areas are considered here: person-centred language and hopeful talk.

Person-centred language

The use of the medicalised language of diagnosis tends to reinforce power differentials and can be unhelpful in many ways, obscuring individuality, stigmatizing, and masking social factors in causation. These "diagnostic narratives of difference and individual deficit" (Johnstone et al., 2018, p. 6) pathologize mental distress, diminishing a person's agency, when it is frequently a "sane reaction to insane circumstances" (Longden, 2013) and understandable when you consider the circumstances that led to it.

So how might this impact mental health nursing practice? Adopting strategies that help people to understand and integrate their meanings of their mental distress is important. The use of diagnostic language closes down possibilities for considering what particular distressing experiences mean and what they might be telling us about what we need to attend to. Consider for example the idea of a "Voice Hearer" versus a "Schizophrenic". A diagnosis of schizophrenia, a contested term that commonly brings negative connotations of chronicity, risk of violence, stigmatizing attitudes, pessimism, and exclusion, is rarely identified with positively (Woods, 2015). The term "Voice Hearer" by comparison has emerged from the Hearing Voices Movement, and is a term that:

> ...points to a distinct but complex aspect of experience without invoking ideas of disease, illness, abnormality, or even distress. If psychiatric labels frequently construe those so diagnosed as objects of medical knowledge and as passive recipients of care, voice-hearers positively claim an identity which signals an affiliation or belonging to a wider community of people who share their experiences and the desire to change negative perceptions and treatments of them.
>
> (Woods, 2015, p. 2387)

In other words, "Voice Hearer" is a term that has been selected and appropriated by those who own the experience and have claimed the right to name it. Woods goes on to discuss the potential beneficial effects of this in terms of helpful responses:

> If we listen, really listen, the statement "I am a voice-hearer" issues a twofold invitation: it asks that we bracket any assumptions about the nature of auditory verbal hallucinations and their status as symptom, and it opens up a space for conversation, a space in which it is not only possible but important to ask about who or what the voices are, what they say, and what meaning they have in the context of a person's sense of self and world. "I am a voice-hearer" might not be an easy thing to hear but the real challenge lies in how you, the clinician, respond.
>
> (Woods, 2015, p. 2387).

We know from research that compares voice hearers who cope well with those who do not, that being able to develop a frame of reference regarding the voices is one of the factors that is important. To be able to do this, voice hearers need to be able to talk about their experiences with someone who is interested in them as a person rather than just as someone with an illness (Romme and Escher, 1989). Also important is finding meaning in the experience. Considering voice hearing in the frame of medical diagnosis, a disorder of the brain, renders such processes invalid. Romme and Escher recommend based on their research that to help people mental health workers need be able to:

- To accept the patient's experience of the voices.
- To try to understand the different language patients use to describe their frame of reference as well as the different language the voices use for communication. Often a world of symbols and feelings is involved. For example, the voices might speak about light and dark when expressing love and aggression.
- To consider helping the individual communicate with the voices. Issues of differentiating good and bad voices and accepting the person's own negative emotions may be involved. Such acceptance may be assisted when support is given to promote self-esteem.
- To stimulate the patient to meet other people with similar experiences and to read about hearing voices in order to diminish the taboo and the isolation. (p. 215)

Doing this means moving away from diagnostic categories and symptomatology and moving towards communication patterns that allow the person's voice to be foregrounded. Consider for example a care plan for a person who has been having troubling voices over a long number of years, despite "antipsychotic" treatment. A key starting point is identification of needs and the development of need statements. If we work from a psychiatric model, a need statement might be:

Noel has a long history of treatment resistant schizophrenia, he suffers with persecutory auditory hallucinations and self-harms regularly. He has been non-compliant with medication recently.

Operating from a person-centred, strengths-based approach that acknowledges the centrality of personal experience, an alternative need statement might state:

Noel hears numerous voices in his head on most days, most of whom say derogatory things about him. They started around the when time when he was bullied in school. They are worse in the evenings when he is alone and not active and get worse whenever he has a row with his mother. They make him feel really scared and bad about himself. He understands them as coming from outside himself, and feels they are very powerful and dangerous. To cope he sometimes shouts back at them but mostly he tries to block them out by playing loud music. This causes trouble with his family. On occasions he cuts himself as the physical pain takes his mind away from the mental distress caused by what they are saying and satisfies their need for him to be punished. He has one good voice who comforts him and tries to help him stand up for himself, this voice he calls "sis". He has chosen not to take his tablets on occasions as the make him feel "distant" from himself and very tired.

The latter statement aims to describe the person's experiences, not simply or entirely in their own words, but using the person's frame of reference and is formulated by what we understand as professionals (informed by evidence generated from research with services users) as being particularly relevant to their particular experiences. Supporting people to move away from identification with stigmatizing diagnostic labels and exploring their own narrative is a key component of professional helping practice. Considering mental health difficulties as "problems of living" (Szasz, 1974) will likely have different consequences for a person compared to having a diagnosis of a disorder. Mental health nurses need to work with people according to the person's frame of reference. Useful also in supporting people to find meaning in their experiences is raising awareness of peer support organizations and activist groups for example Intervoice, Mad in America, or Mental Health Foundation. Working and communicating in this way can have powerful consequences for how families, supporters, and other members of teams make meaning about mental health difficulties. The use of person-centred talk extends to communication with relatives, supports, other staff, and the general public in public and private fora. For example, the use of terms such as "persons with a mental illness" versus "the mentally ill" has been shown to improve tolerance levels amongst the public (Granello and Gibbs, 2016).

Hopeful talk

The rhetoric of "recovery" has become part of the lexicon of terms used in mental health care. This is formalized in government policies and locally in "recovery care plans" and "recovery groups" that aim to offer a more optimistic understanding of mental health problems emphasizing the possibility of recovery, inclusion, and self-determination. The language we use needs to be congruent with a philosophy of recovery; conveying hope, optimism, strength rather than weakness, and emphasizing personal strengths and coping mechanisms. For example, terms such as such as "treatment resistant" and "non-compliant" and "lacking insight", imply the fault lies with the individual and convey pessimistic, judgemental perspectives. Consider for example:

1. Treatment-resistant or The treatment has not helped the person.
2. Non-compliant or The person decided not to take the drugs as the side effects have been too disturbing.
3. Lacks insight or The person has their own understanding of their life and difficulties (as we all have).

The SAFEWARDS project (referred to above), aims to provide a model for understanding and modifying episodes of conflict and containment in psychiatric wards and includes "staff modifiers" as key factors in explaining variance of such episodes. These include how staff interact and communicate with and about patients and the extent to which their communication indicates positive appreciation, compassion, and respect; their skills in dealing with difficult interactions; regulation of their emotional responses; and their understanding of patients' difficulties and behaviours (Bowers, 2014). Through a synthesis of their own and other research the model proposes a range of interventions that have been tested and shown to reduce the frequency of conflict and containment in acute psychiatric wards. Many of the interventions outlined in the SAFEWARDS project involve communication that involves providing narrative with and about service-users that enables them and staff to take ownership of their actions and any associated consequences. This acknowledgement of the power of language in the form of spoken words between individuals that are seeking to understand and express care for each other is central to a person-centred approach. It helps to create a space where the nurse as an expert mental health practitioner is recognising the expertise that resides in the service-user regarding their personhood. It shifts the position of the nurse as a subject who holds expert knowledge about the patient, and "I know best" scenario, to a position of being a skilled communicator whose function is to enable the service-user to articulate, in language, their subjectivity and consequently reduces the needs for distress to escalate into critical incidents. The power balance is redressed through the skilful use of language. For example, one of the interventions is a "Mutual Help Meeting" which involves staff facil-itating a meeting of all services users, preferably every day to allow dis-cussion about how everyone can help everyone else during the day. This supports the idea of service-users having a socially valued role as some who can be helpful and make a meaningful contribution. Another intervention, "Positive Words" involves saying something positive about each patient at the handover. This can relate to a quality they possess or the way in which staff have been able to support them and offering psychological explana-tions for difficult or disruptive behaviour. This is a good example of a strategy aimed at making staff aware of their communication about service-users and adjusting it to ensure that is does not entirely focus on problems, conveying negative perceptions, but instead acknowledges positive elements of the patient's behaviour or experiences. Examples provided by project include expression of an interest in something, coping with some difficulty, enjoying an activity, elements of their personal history, like past roles. "Discharge messages" involves staff facilitating on day of discharge every service-user to write a message for display on the unit about what they liked about the ward, the staff, and their stay together with a positive and helpful piece of advice for new patients. This helps to imbue hope and reinforces the notion of services-users as having agency and valid opinions with something to offer each other in terms of support (Bowers et al., 2011).

Reflection on practice

A practical example of reflection on use of language relates to my clinical practice, working with people who hear voices. The "Maastricht Interview" (MI) is a structured interview which helps a person who hears voices to gain an understanding of the experience of voice hearing in terms of its origins and meaning in their lives (Romme and Escher, 1989). Questions relate to specific details of the voice hearing experience, including for example who the voices are, their characteristics, the person's relationship with them, when they started, coping strategies they employ, and factors that influence them; with the aim of gaining insight into who the voices are, and what function they serve in the person's life. The interview is conducted by a person who has been trained in the approach and results in a report being prepared based on the interview and a construct being developed by the interviewer and the inter-viewee which provides a summary and interpretation of the person's experi-ences. This involves mutual discussion to arrive at a shared understanding.

I worked with a man who has heard many voices, over a 40-year period, which tended to become more troublesome at times in his life where he experienced loss, for example bereavement and loss of autonomy. In preparing the first draft of the report, trying to outline my understanding of his coping strategies, I wrote about what happens when the voices and paranoia that he experiences became overwhelming. I described this as:

> Alan (pseudonym) tends to isolate himself when he finds the voices and the paranoia that they cause him to feel becomes too much.

In accordance with the process of the MI, I gave the draft report to Alan to read, review, and amend. His response in relation to the above statement was that he did not agree with this understanding. The use of the word "isolate", for him, implied something negative, whereas his understanding was that when this situation arose, he "made a decision to spend some time alone".

For Alan this was a positive coping mechanism, which he initiated and had found to be a helpful strategy. This resulted in a discussion about the language that professionals use, how it reveals ways of understanding and the impact this can have on the people we work with, both service users and other staff. Characterizing Alan's response to the distress associated with voice hearing as "isolative" constructs it as a negative response. The inclination to do so stems from a professionalized knowledge of certain behaviours as being "adaptive" or "mal-adaptive". Avoidance of contact with others is understood as one of the negative symptoms of schizophrenia, and one which is considered detrimental to recovery. The effects of this are worthy of reflection. Consider the effect on the voice hearer. The coping strategy (which is one we all commonly employ when things get too much) is now considered part of his symptomatology, another negative in a long line of negatives associated with a diagnosis of schizophrenia. Checking with him and considering the language which emphasizes his choice and personal agency in "making a decision" depicts an adult person taking control of their emotional well-being. Describing the action as "spending some time alone" rather than "isolate" normalizes it as a legitimate response.

The tendency of mental health staff to pathologise human responses is referred to by Allen (1981, p. 357) as "a reformulation in the language of pathology". She noted that the reformulation of events or behaviours as pathologies tended to be preferred over the original description resulting in a foreclosure of the possibility of generating alternative or conflicting interpretations. Psychiatric systems traditionally privilege professional knowledge over service-user knowledge. The Maastricht approach to voice hearing and paranoia is based on an understanding of the voice hearer as being the expert on their own lives. The process of supporting the person to explore their experiences (be it in a group or interview setting) involves a collaboration, where each brings something to the table, but that the voice hearer's experience and understanding is privileged. The important issue here is not a general one regarding whether "deciding to be on your own" is a helpful or unhelpful strategy, the issue is the foregrounding of the person's perspective.

Conclusion

This chapter has considered the way in which the language used by mental health nurses in communication with service-users, their families, the public, and among professional colleagues has important consequences. The use of psychiatrically oriented language and pessimistic talk produces versions of reality that are unhelpful for service-users. Moving towards communication patterns that allow the person's voice to be foregrounded and language congruent with a philosophy of recovery that conveys hope and optimism, emphasizing personal strengths rather than weakness involves skilled communication and redresses power balance in the nursing/service-user relationship. Reflection on practice should include a consideration of language. To conclude, I offer several practical tips for improving communication in Box 10.1.

Box 10.1   Practical tips

Practical tips for improving communication

- Avoid use of medicalized language in communication with and about service-users.
- Foreground and value the person's frame of reference by exploring, recording, and communicating the person's experience in rich detail.
- Reflect on the language you use and the extent to which it conveys meaning, hope, and optimism.

References

Allen, H., 1981. "Voices of concern": A study of verbal communication about patients in a psychiatric day unit. *J. Adv. Nurs. 6*, 355–362.

Allen, R., Nairn, R., 1997. Media depictions of mental illness: an analysis of the use of dangerousness. *Aust. N. Z. J. Psychiatry 31* (3), 375–381.

Angermeyer, M., Dietrich, S., Pott, D., Matschinger, H., 2005. Media consumption and desire for social distance towards people with schizophrenia. *Eur. Psychiatry 20* (3), 246–250.

Bilić, B., Georgaca, E., 2007. Representations of mental Illness in Serbian newspapers: A critical discourse analysis. *Qualit. Res. Psychol. 4* (1–2), 67–186.

Bowers, L., 2014. Safewards: A new model of conflict and containment on psychiatric wards. *J. Psychiatr. Ment. Health Nurs. 29* (2), 331–340.

Bowers, L., Stewart, D., Papadopoulos, C., Dack, C., Ross, J., Khanom, H., Jeffrey, D., 2011. *In-patient Violence and Aggression: A Literature Review*. Institute of Psychiatry at the Maudsely and King's College, London.

Charland, L., 2004. A madness for identity: psychiatric labels, consumer autonomy, and the perils of the internet. *Philos. Psychiatry Psychol. 11* (4), 335–349.

Cheek, J., Rudge, T., 1993. The power of normalisation: Foucauldian perspectives on contemporary Australian health care practices. *Aust. J. Soc. Issues 28* (4), 271–284.

Cheek, J., Rudge, T., 1994a. Nursing as textually mediated reality. *Nurs. Inq. 1*, 15–22.

Cheek, J., Rudge, T., 1994b. Webs of documentation: The dis-course of case notes. *Aust. J. Commun. 21* (2), 41–52.

Coverdale, J., Nairn, R., Claasen, D., 2002. Depictions of mental illness in print media: A prospective national sample. *Aust. N. Z. J. Psychiatry 36* (5), 697–700.

Crowe, M., 2000. Constructing normality: A discourse analysis of the DSM-IV. *J. Psychiatr. Ment. Health Nurs. 7*, 69–77.

Daniel Yanklovich Group Inc., 1990. *Public Attitudes Towards People with Chronic Mental Illness*. Author, Boston, MA.

Diefenbach, D., 1997. The portrayal of mental illness on prime-time television. *J. Commun. Psychol. 25* (3), 289–302.

Dietrich, S., Heider, D., Matschinger, H., Angermeyer, M., 2006. Influence of newspaper reporting on adolescents' attitudes toward people with mental illness. *Soc. Psychiatry Psychiatr. Epidemiol. 41* (4), 318–322.

Dyson, H., Gorvin, L., 2017. How is a label of borderline personality disorder constructed on Twitter: A critical discourse analysis. *Issues Men. Health Nurs. 38* (10), 780–790.

Farrelly, M. (2015) The discursive construction of mental health problems in Irish print news media. Ph.D. dissertation. Dublin City University, Dublin. http://doras.dcu.ie/20763/ (accessed 09.11.2020).

Francis, C., Pirkis, J., Blood, R., Dunt, D., Burgess, P., Morley, B., Stewart, A., Putnis, P., 2004. The portrayal of mental health and illness in Australian non-fiction media. *Aust. N. Z. J. Psychiatry 38* (7), 541–546.

Gerbner, G., Gross, L., Morgan, M., Signorielli, N., 1986. Living with television: The dynamics of the cultivation process. In: Bryant, J., Zillman, D. (Eds.), *Perspectives on Media Effects*. Lawrence Erlbaum, Hilldale, NJ, pp. 17–40.

Giles, D., Newbold, J., 2011. Self-and other-diagnosis in user-led mental health online communities. *Qual. Health Res. 21* (3), 419–428.

Granello, D., Gibbs, T., 2016. The power of language and labels: "The mentally ill" versus "people with mental illnesses". *J. Couns. Dev. 94* (1), 31–40.

Granello, D., Pauley, P., Carmichael, A., 1999. Relationship of the media to attitudes toward people with mental illness. *J. Hum. Couns. Educ. Dev. 38* (2), 98–110.

Hazelton, M., 1997. Reporting mental health: A discourse analysis of mental health related newspapers in two Australian newspapers. *Aust. N. Z. J. Psychiatry 6* (2), 73–89.

Irving, K., Treacy, M., Scott, A., Hyde, A., Butler, M., Mc Neela, P., 2006. Discursive practice in the documentation of patients' assessments. *J. Adv. Nurs. 53* (2), 151–159.

Johnstone, L., Boyle, M., Cromby, J., Dillon, J., Harper, D., Kinderman, P., Longden, E., Pilgrim, D., Read, J., 2018. *The Power Threat Meaning Framework: Towards the Identification of Patterns in Emotional Distress, Unusual Experiences and Troubled or Troubling Behaviour, as an Alternative to Functional Psychiatric Diagnosis.* British Psychological Society, Leicester.

Longden, E., 2013. *Learning from the Voices in My Head.* TED Books 39, New York.

McGinty, E., Webster, D., Jarlenski, M., Barry, C., 2014. News media framing of serious mental illness and gun violence in the United States, 1997–2012. *Am. J. Public Health 104* (3), 406–413.

Millar, R., Sands, N., 2010. "He did what? Well that wasn't handed over!" Communicating risk in mental health. *J. Psychiatr. Ment. Health Nurs. 20*, 345–354.

Moncrieff, J., 2010. Psychiatric diagnosis as a political device. *Soc. Theory Health 8* (4), 370–382.

Moore, G., 2017. Critical incidents in mental health units may be better understood and managed with a Freudian/Lacanian psychoanalytic framework. *Eur. J. Psychother. Couns. 19* (1), 43–60.

Morgan, A., Jorm, A., 2009. Recall of news stories about mental illness by Australian youth: Associations with help-seeking attitudes and stigma. *Aust. N. Z. J. Psychiatry 43* (9), 866–872.

Nairn, R., Coverdale, J., Claasen, D., 2001. From source material to news story in New Zealand print media: A prospective study of the stigmatizing processes in depicting mental illness. *Aust. N. Z. J. Psychiatry 35* (5), 654–659.

Pantnic, I., 2014. Online social networking and mental health. *Cyberpsychol. Behav. Soc. Netw. 17* (10), 652–657.

Penn, D., Chamberlin, C., Mueser, K., 2003. The effects of a documentary film about schizophrenia on psychiatric stigma. *Schizophr. Bull. 29* (2), 383–391.

Philo, G., Henderson, L., McCracken, K., 2010. *Making a Drama Out of a Crisis: Authentic Portrayals of Mental Illness in TV Drama.* SHIFT/Department of Health, London.

Romme, M., Escher, A., 1989. Hearing voices. *Schizophr. Bull. 15* (2), 209–216.

Stout, P., Villegas, J., Jennings, N., 2004. Images of mental illness in the media: Identifying gaps in the research. *Schizophr. Bull. 30* (3), 543–561.

Szasz, T., 1974. The Myth of Mental Illness. Harper Collins, New York.

Thornton, J., Wahl, O., 1996. Impact of a newspaper articles on attitudes toward mental illness. *Journal of Community Psychology 24* (1), 17–25.

Wahl, O., Roth, R., 1982. Television images of mental illness: results of a Metropolitan Washington Media Watch. *Journal of Broadcasting 26* (2), 599–605.

Wilson, C., Nairn, R., Coverdale, J., Panapa, A., 1999a. Constructing mental illness as dangerous: A pilot study. *Aust. N. Z. J. Psychiatry 33* (2), 240–247.

Wilson, C., Nairn, R., Coverdale, J., Panapa, A., 1999b. Mental illness depictions in prime-time drama: Identifying the discursive resources. *Aust. N. Z. J. Psychiatry 33* (2), 32–239.

Woods, A., 2015. The art of medicine. Voices, identity, and meaning-making. *The Lancet 386*, 2386–2387.

Chapter 11

Exploring the "talk" of suicide

Using discourse-informed approaches in exploring suicide risk

Andrew Reeves

Practitioner highlights

From this chapter, there are six core practitioner messages:

- It is critical for practitioners to consider both professional and personal challenges when working with suicide, to support effective communication.
- Predominant mental health practice around working with risk tends to favour a risk factor approach. While this is helpful to an extent, it should not replace effective communication.
- Practitioners can be fearful of asking clients about suicide, retreating into predominantly reflective responses rather than more explicit, explorative ones.
- Asking open, empathic, and clear questions about suicide does not prompt its likelihood, but instead can be an important factor in reducing risk.
- Effective communication facilitates both practitioner and client understanding of suicidal thinking. A client is likely more able to talk openly about their suicidal thoughts where they experience the therapist to be compassionate and non-judgemental.
- Human relationships, and clear communications, are the critical cornerstones of work with suicidal clients.

Introduction

It is an interesting paradox that for many who train in the helping professions: social work, counselling, psychotherapy, occupational therapy, and so on, the time spent on how they might most effectively respond to their clients or patients who are suicidal (herein after referred to as "clients") is disproportionately low by comparison to the number of clients they are likely to see who present with some degree of suicide risk. That is, despite that the presentation of suicide risk of some degree is relatively common in practice, we are often ill-equipped by our training experiences to respond to it (see also Kiyimba et al., this volume). Albeit some time ago now, I undertook a questionnaire study looking at how trainees on British Association for Counselling and Psychotherapy (BACP) Accredited training courses dealt with issues of risk in their training. Amongst several findings was the outcome that nearly 10% of Programme Leaders did not feel their graduates – counsellors and psychotherapists – were adequately prepared to work with suicidal clients.

Over the years, and as a consequence of the suicide of one of my own clients in therapy (which I discuss later), I have written about working with suicide extensively and trained many thousands of mental health practitioners in ways of working with suicide potential. It is probably fair to say there is not a shortage of risk assessment training sessions to attend but, as we will explore, very few focus on the dialogic mechanisms of effective work and instead look at the application of "science" – the risk assessment tools and tick boxes – to the task of prediction. It seems anathematic to me that the energy invested in the science of risk assessment is, typically, at the expense of dialogic risk exploration; that we may understand more about an individual's self-annihilatory experiences through the ticking of some boxes rather than asking them about how they feel. This too has been the experience of many of the attendees to my training sessions.

It is my intention in this chapter therefore, to unpack some of the myths around working with suicidal clients, including the faith given to the risk assessment tools, and argue instead for a turn back to discourse. This is not without challenge however, as a dialogic approach to working with suicide risk demands things of the practitioner: to be truly present in the suicide shared-narrative, the practitioner but be prepared to go to difficult places with their client and understand what it is in themselves they bring along in that process. Perhaps it is this personal/professional demand of dialogic work with risk that leads many to retreat to the relative safety of the tick box?

The challenges of working with suicidal clients

The challenges of working with suicidal clients are multi-faceted and can, at a most basic level, be divided across a professional and personal frame. This, of course, does not do full justice to the complexities that can be encountered, inter- and intra-personally when working with suicide risk, but a consideration of the personal and professional aspects is an important starting point for most practitioners. It is critical that such challenges are outlined and explored because, as outlined previously, a dialogic approach to working with risk demands that the practitioner has some insight into their own professional and personal responses, to support the potential intimacy of the narrative.

Professional

There are several professional factors that will be present when working with suicide potential; these include:

- Managing expectations of confidentiality
- Understanding the different ways in which suicide may present
- Fear of "getting it wrong"
- Translating risk in a multi-disciplinary context
- A careful balance of policy, practice, ethics, and values

Managing expectations of confidentiality

Most practitioners will work to some form of confidentiality agreement, typically outlined in a contract agreed with the client from the outset. This will be the case for those working across a range of settings, such as statutory settings (health and social care, for example), education (schools, colleges, and universities), third sector settings, and independent (private) practice, for example. While the contract will attend to various practical factors, it also outlines how confidentiality, including that of risk to self (suicide potential or self-injury) will be responded to.

While some independent practitioners may hold confidentiality in the face of suicide risk, most organisational settings, and most independent practitioners will limit confidentiality should they believe their client presents with an immediate suicide risk. While many practitioners will routinely make these agreements, fewer actively consider the ramifications of them: how will *immediacy* of risk be measured? Many clients will explore suicidal ideation in helping relationships (thoughts of suicide, rather than an intent to act on those thoughts), but this would not constitute an immediate risk and many practitioners would hold their client's confidentiality to allow for exploration of such thoughts. Herein lies a truth spoken by Shneidman (1998) when he wrote, "Most people who commit suicide talk about it; most people who talk about suicide do not commit it. Which to believe?" Making judgements about the intent of another, and particularly around whether they are focussed on ending their own life, can feel onerous judgements indeed.

Understanding the different ways in which suicide may present

While suicide can be defined simply as "the act of killing yourself" (American Psychological Association 2020), the process of *being suicidal* can be highly complex and individual. There are many theories that offer some understanding of a move towards suicide (Shneidman, 1998; Joiner, 2005; O'Conner et al., 2011). My own research, based on a critical discourse analysis (Reeves et al., 2006) identified three primary interpretive repertoires around suicide:

- Suicide ends existential crisis:
  "What's the point, what's the point in carrying on? I feel really alone with it all ... I just feel that I don't exist – I don't belong in the life I live in...".
- Suicide removes a sense of being "stuck" with the negotiations and manoeuvrings of life:
  "I'm thinking about stopping it. I don't see what keeping me here, or why I carry on. I feel stuck and cannot see a way forward. I need to get out and go somewhere else – I need to get out of peoples way and get out of this stuckness".
- Suicide ends apathy and fatigue generated by the burdensome nature of life:
  "I just feel too tired to carry on. It feels so heavy, I don't know if I can continue to manage it any longer/further. I feel so tired and exhausted in keeping it going. I don't want people to worry about me anymore. I need to take the pain away – to ease the pain".

These different intrapersonal drivers for suicide are further complicated by behavioural presentation. That is, suicide is often considered as a slow move towards death, perhaps following a trauma or as a consequence of physical illness, with the person putting their affairs in order, perhaps writing suicide notes, and so on. While this is certainly true for many, it does not capture others' experience, which can include living with the thoughts of suicide on a daily basis, through to not having suicidal thoughts but responding to a crisis with an impulsive act. This can be captured in Figure 11.1. Living with suicidal thoughts daily, a move towards suicide or an impulsive act each presents different challenges to the practitioner.

Fear of "getting it wrong"

In considering the management of the contract, in the context of the complex way in which suicide might present intra-personally, cognitively, in-terpersonally, and behaviourally, understandably leaves many practitioners fearful of "getting it wrong" (Reeves and Mintz, 2001). Of the research

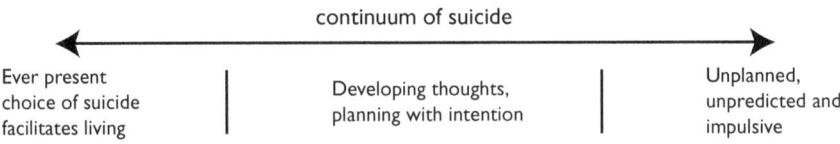

Figure 11.1 The continuum of suicidal action.

available exploring the demands of working with suicidal clients in helping relationships (of which there is surprisingly little), the fear of getting it wrong – of either breaking confidentiality unnecessarily, or not acting in response to concerns with a subsequent suicide, can haunt many practitioners in their daily work. The fear has often been described as immobilizing, leading to practitioners avoiding discussions about suicide, where possible, through to the impact of vicarious trauma. It is noted in the research that ongoing work with suicide potential can be as impactful, psychologically and emotionally, on the practitioner as experiencing the death of a client through suicide.

Communicating risk in a multi-disciplinary context

While this is not the case across the board, many practitioners are based within multi-disciplinary teams, where interventions are informed through an array of different, and sometimes competing or contradictory, theoretical, and philosophical lenses. Finding a common language through which client experience can be understood and, where necessary, shared, can be a significant hurdle. In the context of working with suicide potential, increasingly the shared language has been through the "reading" of risk assessment tools and the interpretation of such data. The dialogic interpretation of a client's experience, often in the face of science, is pushed down the pecking order. Communicating concern to others, or indeed supporting ongoing work in the face of perceived risk, can be difficult when the data speaks otherwise.

A careful balance of policy, practice, ethics, and values

Overall therefore, practitioners professionally navigate their way through a difficult terrain of: policy expectations; practice parameters; the interpretation and application of various "ethical frameworks" and good practice guidance; as well as their own values they have often worked tirelessly to embed in their own work. It is not uncommon for such values to sit at odds with the expectation of policy that, in turn, adds to the personal challenges to be considered.

Personal

In addition to the professional factors, some of which have been outlined above, are the personal ones. Many writers in counselling and psychotherapy argue that the therapist should 'leave themselves at the door' of the therapy room. While this expectation might be theoretically more consistent with some schools of therapy, for example, psychoanalysis, the reality might instead be argued that no practitioner, regardless of their theoretical orientation, can ever be truly objective in a helping relationship and therefore, the subjective experience of the practitioner will inevitably be present. In this context, there are some specific personal challenges practitioner will need to address:

- Personal experiences of mental health crisis
- Personal views in relation to suicide
- The degree of dissonance with agency policy
- Self-care and ongoing coping strategies

Personal experiences of mental health crisis

While some would have us believe that there are people who experience mental health difficulties, and then there are the rest of us who are, presumably, "sorted", this is, of course, nonsense. In the same way we all have our physical health to attend to, which might include being well, temporarily impaired or struggling with longer-term conditions, the same is true for our mental health. In that frame therefore, the practitioner's own experience of mental health difficulties and how they have been able to navigate them – through their own support and/or help from others – will play an important role in shaping how they respond to mental health distress in others. Specifically, the extent to which the practitioner can find a narrative for their distress, again, either for themselves or for sharing with others, will be important here too. Put simply, if we have been able make sense of our own distress through self-talk, or by talking with others, that is more likely to position us to provide that space with our clients.

The concept of the "wounded healer" (Larisey, 2012) is well established: that those who find their way into helping professional roles do so, at least in part, because of their own previous "wounds". It is not uncommon however, drawing anecdotally over 30 years of practice and support by some limited research evidence (Adams, 2013), that helpers often struggle to be helped themselves. Relationally therefore, one might speculate, as to the impact of a helper who struggles to verbalise their own distress on their capacity to support another do the same.

Personal views in relation to suicide

Suicide is one of those topics that is rarely viewed through a neutral lens; people can often have a visceral response to suicide, in the same way they can about death more generally. The narrative mechanisms developed through social story-telling to soften the truth of death are everyday apparent: going to sleep; being at rest; passing on; and so on. Add into the mix the stigma that still surrounds mental health – albeit to a lesser extent recently perhaps – and certainly the historical echoes of the shame of suicide when it was seen to be "against God", or an illegal act, still abound.

Practitioners are not tabula rasa when it comes to suicide therefore, and their personal views about suicide – ranging from believing people have a right to end their own life if they have the capacity to make that decision, through to the choice of suicide never being acceptable – will be present in the helping relationship, explicitly or implicitly. Such views will be shaped by a range of factors, such as: faith; music; literature; experiences of suicide personally or amongst family and friends; training, and so on. The challenge is for the practitioner to be willing to engage with an internal reflection so that their views are known to them and held accordingly in the helping relationship so that they do not consciously, or unconsciously, shape the nature of the help being offered. Supervision, which is discussed in a little more detail later (and in Helps, this volume), is important here in helping practitioners to reflect on their own philosophical, practical, and theoretical relationship to suicide. Important here is Shea's (2011, p. 4) observations that,

> ... when a [practitioner] begins to understand his or her own attitudes, biases, and responses to suicide, he or she can become more psychologically and emotionally available to a suicidal client. Clients seem to be able to sense when a [practitioner] is comfortable with the topic of suicide. At that point, and with such a [practitioner], clients may feel safe enough to share the immediacy of their pull towards death.

The degree of dissonance with agency policy

In the light of personal experiences of mental health crisis, and personal views about suicide, it is not uncommon for practitioners to find themselves working in settings where their personal views are contradictory with those of the agency. This has to be professionally managed, with practitioners sometimes having to act in a way inconsistent with how they might personally. My own research amongst counsellors suggested however, that when there was a conflict between a counsellor's own view of suicide and that of the agency within which the work was taking place, they tended to favour their own view, disregarding that of the agency (Reeves and Mintz, 2001). This, of course, raises some difficult professional and ethical questions.

Self-care and ongoing coping strategies

It is an ethical requirement of most commonly referred to ethical frameworks for practitioners to pay explicit reference to their own well-being and self-care. Formal supervisory arrangements, again often a requirement of professional bodies for many different professions, play an important role in ensuring the restorative care of the practitioner. Beyond such formal arrangements however, it is imperative the practitioner puts in place their own strategies for self-care. Failure to do so often leads to vicarious trauma, compassion fatigue and burnout (Marriage and Marriage, 2005; Moore and Donohue, 2016). Helping professionals are not immune to the dangers of dissociation, where the felt experience of the helping relationship is lost to a sense of attack, anger and resentment of clients who are perceived to be "too needy" or "manipulative". In this context, the capacity for an empathic and meaningful narrative is lost.

Research insights and the evidence base

The literature on working with suicide is extensive, but also limited too. Extensive insofar as the search for a definitive answer to the question, *who is most likely to end their life through suicide* seems to lead to an insatiable quest and endless studies. In writing this chapter I undertook a brief literature search of academic papers related to the search terms "suicide risk assessment", since 2019, and returned in the region of 17,200 papers. Of those reviewed, the majority attended to one of the following predominant themes:

- The broad identification of specific risk factors
- The delivery of suicide intervention programmes
- Understanding suicide across different demographic and cultural groups
- The epidemiology of suicide
- Models of suicide thinking and pre-suicidal process
- The development, implementation and evaluation of suicide risk assessment tools

Space does not allow for a meaningful account of the extent of literature here; rather, and perhaps more importantly, is a consideration of what might be missing. In that context it is helpful to consider the meta-analysis, conducted by Large et al. (2016), cited in Reeves (2017), who stated,

> *that 95% of high-risk patients do not die through suicide, and that there had been no meaningful increase in the accuracy of prediction of suicide over the last 40 years.*

Reeves (2019, p. 3) goes on to state that suicide risk assessment tools,

> *may contribute to an understanding [of suicide risk] and may give permission for more of an exploration, but the problem is that too many view them as the 'start and stop' of working with suicide, rather than simply a starting point. We place so much trust in their predictive accuracy that, too often, we forget to turn back to the client.*

The Zero Target for suicide in the UK in National Health Service (NHS) settings (Deputy Prime Minister's Office, 2015) is predicated on the assumption that enough is known of the *who* and *how* of suicide that such targets become not only aspirational, but instead achievable. Whereas, looking back at Large et al's assertion, the *who* and *how* continue to be elusive concepts that set up false expectations for policy makers, researchers, practitioners, and, perhaps, clients too.

Related to these epistemological and ontological conundrums with respect to suicide, is the place of communication. As asserted elsewhere in this chapter, we too often rely on the efficacy of risk assessment tools for fear of going to a more frightening place. I offer a personal reflection here.

Reflections on the science

I mentioned previously the death of my client early on in my career and the traumatic impact that had on me. By traumatic impact, I refer to trauma with a capital T, as opposed to it simply being distressing. I became hypervigilant to potential risk, experienced flashbacks, nightmares etc., and stepped away from practise for a while to allow for a period of recovery. Embarking on my own doctoral studies in this area, my research proposal to an established UK university was the development of a short-risk assessment tool for humanistic counsellors that would, when completed with clients, definitively tell the practitioner whether the client was going to kill themselves. Needless to say, the University enthusiastically bit my hand off and invited me to study there.

It was only during my doctorate that the reflective penny finally dropped: such a tool did not exist, but I had wanted it to because of my trauma following my client's death and, simply, never wanting to go there again. I had lost the capacity of working with uncertainty, which remains the cornerstone of practice with suicide potential. On this realization my research took a very different turn – a turn to discourse – and looked at ways in which practitioners might be supported, through training, to sit with uncertainty too, while building confidence and capacity to talk to clients about suicide. My anxiety, which drove me initially to undertake the development of a risk assessment tool was neatly captured by one of my latter participants, who insightfully said as part of a feedback session,

> "*I was wondering, is this a personal journey, are you Sir Galahad on his horse riding out to save the nation because you felt such a failure in yourself. And I wondered about that. I didn't in any way feel judgmental I just felt, oh, what's that about. This poor man has to tell the nation, to protect the nation…*". *She continued, "What I was left with was the fact that it was something that you were passionate about … which is a strange use of words … but from your experience you had been through with your client, you didn't want any of us … you were quite protective … you didn't want any of us going through what you had been through.*"

That sense of "failure in yourself" poignantly captured that fear of getting it wrong. As one therapist once said to me, the feared perception from others is that "good enough therapists keep their clients alive"; even acknowledging the ridiculous nature of this comment, deep down the fear might be of it being a truth.

The importance of discourse

The central assertion here of this chapter is of the critical importance of effective communication with clients at risk of suicide that transcends the two-dimensional nature of a risk assessment tool or questionnaire. The explorative nature of communication not only provides the best opportunity for the practitioner – and more importantly, the client – with an opportunity of sense-making in relation to suicidal thinking, but also creates further opportunities for deeper exploration and helps position the client with greater opportunities for change. Discourse, in of itself, will not prevent suicide; it will, however, provide the narrative space for suicide to be explored in a meaningful way. Revisiting the work of Schneidman (1996, p. 6), he asserts,

> ... our best route to understanding suicide is not through the study of the structure of the brain, nor the study of social statistics, nor the study of mental diseases, but directly through the study of human emotions described ... in the words of the suicidal person. The most important question to a potentially suicidal person is not an inquiry about family history or laboratory tests of blood or spinal fluid, but "where do you hurt?" and "how can I help you?"

Exploring the "where do you hurt and how can I help you" is not a straightforward endeavour, however. In my own critical discourse analysis (Reeves et al., 2006), many practitioner–client assessment transcripts were analysed. They key findings of this study were that:

- Suicide is often not disclosed explicitly by clients – at first mention – and is typically talked about implicitly using metaphor, e.g., "I wish I could get out of everyone's way"
- At the first reference to suicide by the client, practitioners – regardless of theoretical orientation – tend to revert to reflective responses rather than explorative ones, e.g., "So it seems as if ... I hear that ... you are saying that ..."
- The predominant use of reflective responses following an implicit reference by a client to suicide typically hinders exploration, as the practitioner becomes defined in the dialogue by the client's position, rather than enabling any meaningful dialogic shift, e.g., [client] "It just goes round and round in my head and I can't seem to find a way

forward"; [practitioner] "You feel really stuck – round and round – and you can't find a way forward". Both client and practitioner get stuck in the "round and round" metaphor, both defining each other and neither finding a way forward

- Practitioners are often fearful of naming suicide – of making the implicit, explicit – for fear of "getting it wrong" or putting the thought into the client's mind: explicit exploration becomes a feared prompt for suicide, where there is no evidence to support this. As institutions and individuals perhaps retreat into risk assessment tools to avoid the relational, practitioners retreat into the reflective to avoid the exploration.

This study, in itself a little dated now, has been replicated by me (unpublished), additionally focusing on working with young people. Even with intervening research, the findings were the same. The implications of avoiding an open communication around suicide with clients is that a number of professional responsibilities are more difficult to meet: the appropriate management of the contract of confidentiality; maintaining work consistent with procedural expectations of the organisation; consistent work with legal and ethical expectations; and missed opportunities for greater therapeutic exploration. The personal implications are often an increased sense of anxiety and a greater propensity to burnout.

Reflections on client work

Research aside, this chapter is fundamentally based on my experiences of working with people who are suicidal, which I have been undertaking for 30 years. I have experienced several client suicides across that time, each one impacting on me professionally and personally in a different way; ranging from an early traumatic response I experienced following the death of a client through suicide soon after a completed counselling session while I was a trainee, through an end-of-life suicide that had been communicated by the individual to all those involved in his care. I will offer an account of some work with a client, who I will call Jake, to illustrate some of challenges raised "in action". Sufficient details of Jake's story have been changed (as well as his name) to protect identity, as well as to illustrate some of the wider issues, not all of which were present in the original work.

Introducing Jake

Jake is 19 years old and comes to see me in a third sector setting for young people. He is well-dressed, articulate and thoughtful. He is seeking out counselling he says, because he is feeling "crap" and it has been like this for some time. He tells me he lives with his mother, who is very supportive, his father having left the family home many years before. He lives with his younger sister but has no contact now with his father. He tells me he specifically wants to see a male therapist because there are no men in his life he can talk to. As the agency requires, he has completed an assessment form before seeing me, which includes questions about risk. He has scored zero on risk, indicating no thoughts of suicide and self-harm.

We begin the session with introductions, and I invite Jake to tell me his story, which he does. It is a sad story of loss – a grief and anger for his missing father; the death through an accident of a friend 4 years previously; and his overwhelming sense of loneliness, of truly being on his own in the world. He tells me that while he loves his family dearly, he could never talk of his feelings with them "because guys just don't do that, people just don't understand". He is lost, adrift, and struggles to find his words.

Early responses to Jake

I am struck by the paradox of Jake: of someone so strong outwardly, yet so young inside and struggling with a searing distress. Also, of someone wanting to be heard, but having been taught that male words for feelings are not acceptable. I must tread warily because if I expect too much from him too soon, he might not return. I must find his language of strength while, at the same time, offering an implicit permission to speak of himself.

I ask him about this assessment form and note, given how he is feeling, he has indicated he does not feel suicidal. I am tentative here, but it also strikes me that suicidal thoughts might well be present for him. He nods and says "yes, that's not an issue for me". I want to be reassured but I am not. But I have asked the question and, in doing so, am hoping I have opened a door if he ever wishes to walk through it.

Subsequent sessions with Jake

We get on well and he comes to the next, and subsequent sessions. I have found a shared humour, and we laugh a lot. I feel a little guilty about whether I am colluding with an avoidance of his feelings, but the laughter feels relational and intimate and a bridge across which we have found a mechanism to truly speak to each other. Then he stops laughing and the eye contact breaks. He says that I asked him a couple of weeks ago about suicide, and he said he was okay. I say yes, I remember. He says he is not okay and thinks of suicide often; he feels that no one would miss him, even though he knows they would.

I am tempted to refer back to his strengths, but see that Jake has said the unsayable and I must be brave and stay with this uncertainty. I acknowledge what he has said but it does not feel enough. I say "How much have you thought about killing yourself Jake? Have you thought about what you would do?" It feels brutal, to the point and I know the phrase "killing yourself" was not his phrase. But I also remember how easy it is to not say the difficult things and, in avoiding them, take Jake away from them too. I am metaphorically holding my breath, wondering if I might have prompted him into thinking more, leading him to the edge. He says no, he hasn't got that far, but he is pleased he has told me. Me asking him so straightforwardly at the beginning did not make him think about suicide, but did enable him to think about his suicidal thoughts – if I know what he means. I say I do; he begins to cry, and I feel terribly sad too. We talk a lot about suicide, and it seems now the door has been opened, all sorts of things can now be talked about. He talks of shame, of having previously been silenced, of hurt, and of not knowing how to live, rather than wanting to die. It strikes me how closely liberation and annihilation can often sit so closely together.

Further reflections

Jake and I worked together over several months and, in that time, his thoughts of suicide ebbed and flowed, like some terrible tide he sometimes wanted to avoid bathing in, but at other times needed to immerse himself in. It would have been so easy from the outset not to have asked Jake about suicide, given his negligible scores on the tick box tools. But I also remind myself that it is often the task of the practitioner to name the difficult things, knowing that the client will decide whether to go there or not. I am also reminded of the big myth about suicide: that by asking about it we might prompt the thought in the other's mind. I know that is not the case, in that asking about suicide, at worst, will leave the level of risk unchanged. At best, it will provide an opportunity to talk about it and, in doing so, the risk of acting on the thoughts can be diminished. I was further reminded too that there isn't a suicidal "type", as Leenaars (1994) calls it, the "bump on the head" (p. 90) that is the definitive indicator of the person who is likely to end their life by suicide. Rather, in moments of crisis or despair, we all have that potential.

Good practice indicators

Drawing together the threads from this chapter, we are able identify some key good practice indicators that can support our communications with people at risk of suicide. To reiterate, the tick box approach to suicide risk assessment is not all bad: such tools can be helpful, but generally in providing a structure through which dialogue can be initiated and explored. The assertion here, and reflecting on Large et al.'s (2016) conclusions, is that risk assessment tools will not offer what we hope of them: a definitive answer, or indeed a good indication, of whether someone is at risk of suicide; it always comes back to the dialogue and how we can support ourselves in the relational process of communication.

Box 11.1   Practical tips

Practical tips for improving communication

- Understand the policy and expectations of the setting.
- Contract carefully and clearly, making clear reference to suicide while considering its potential in the context of the client's narrative.
- It is important to know the higher-risk groups, but this information only informs dialogue, rather than answers, questions.
- Know the warning signs.
- Be able to identify the protective factors and help the client name them.
- Be willing to explore through open and direct questions: Have you ever thought of hurting yourself when you feel bad, or have thoughts of not wanting to be alive anymore?
- Balance both risk factors and protective factors.
- Discuss with supervisor/colleagues/manager, where appropriate.
- Record concerns and actions carefully.
- Obtain consent, where possible, if you need to discuss your concerns with someone else.
- If in doubt about immediate safety, act.

The following practical tips in Box 11.1 for improving communication with people at risk of suicide are, in part, directly related to the discourse and, in part, related to those factors that support discourse. In working with suicide potential, communication does not take place in a vacuum: the professional and personal factors discussed previously need to be addressed fully, carefully, and with due reflection to ensure the discourse is direct, clear, respectful, honest, empathic, and honours the nature of the helping relationship.

Summary

This chapter has maintained a central assertion as to the critical importance of effective communication, rooted in a relational approach, with clients presenting at risk of suicide. Various professional and personal aspects pertinent to effective communication have been highlighted, with a supporting discussion of the importance of discourse in the context of the literature that largely ignores it. Reflections from some sessions with a suicidal client, Jake, have been offered, together with some top tips for effective communication in this frame. One practitioner, when interviewed by me, said that "working with suicide demands that you be brave; be willing to go there". The paradox is that the more suicide is brought into the helping process, the less frightening it can become for both practitioner and client; that effective communication not only enables greater insight but can be a critical holding process at a time of challenge.

References

Adams, M., 2013. *The Myth of the Untroubled Therapist*. Routledge, London.

American Psychological Association, 2020. *Suicide. APA, Washington DC.* https://www.apa.org/topics/suicide/ (accessed 22.11.2020).

Deputy Prime Minister's Office, 2015. *Nick Clegg calls for new ambition for zero suicides across the NHS.* https://www.gov.uk/government/news/nick-clegg-calls-for-zero-suicides-across-the-nhs (accessed 11.2020).

Joiner, T., 2005. *Why People Die by Suicide*. Harvard University Press, Cambridge, MA.

Larisey, K., 2012. *The wounded healer: A Jungian perspective.* http://www.jungatlanta.com/articles/fall12-wounded-healer.pdf (accessed 22.06.2020).

Leenaars, A.A., 1994. *Psychotherapy with suicidal people – a person-centred approach*. Wiley, London.

Marriage, S., Marriage, K., 2005. Too many sad stories: Clinical stress and coping. *Canadian Child and Adolescent Psychiatric Review* 14 (4), 114–117.

Moore, H., Donohue, G., 2016. The impact of suicide prevention on experienced Irish clinicians. *Counselling and Psychotherapy Research* 16 (1), 24–34.

O'Conner, R.C., Cleare, S., Eschle, S., Wetherall, K., Kirtley, O.J., 2011. Towards an integrated motivational–volitional model of suicidal behaviour. In: O'Conner, R.C., Platt, S., Gordon, J. (Eds.), *International Handbook of Suicide Prevention: Research, Policy and Practice*. Wiley, London, pp. 220–240.

Reeves, A., 2017. In a search for meaning: Challenging the accepted know-how of working with suicide risk. *British Journal of Guidance and Counselling* 45 (5), 606–609.

Reeves, A., Bowl, R., Wheeler, S., Guthrie, E., 2006. The hardest words: Exploring the dialogue of suicide in the counselling process – A discourse analysis. *Counselling and Psychotherapy Research* 4 (1), 62–71.

Reeves, A., Mintz, R., 2001. Counsellors' experiences of working with suicidal clients: An exploratory study. *Counselling and Psychotherapy Research* 1 (3), 172–176.

Shea, S.C., 2011. *The Practical Art of Suicide Assessment*. Wiley, London.

Shneidman, E.S., 1998. *The Suicidal Mind*. Oxford University Press, Oxford.

Part III

Learning journeys

From theory to practice

Chapter 12

A PhD learning journey

The value of conversation analysis and discourse approaches for speech and language clinical practice

Alison Drewett

Introduction: Conversation analysis and speech and language therapy

Unsurprisingly, as a speech and language therapist (SLT) I have an interest in language, communication, and talk in general. I am fascinated with how we make connections with people through talk and how talk mediates our friendships, professional relationships, and family interactions. As a mature speech and language therapy student with a background in sociology, I learnt that in principle our professional practice was rooted in both a medical and social model, that viewed individuals in a biopsychosocial perspective. However, much of the focus was firmly on speech and language as opposed to communication, and often if felt more on physiological or neurological ways of thinking to understand human communication. Even linguistic courses were mainly based on idealized social situations often, depicting language sequences divorced from real talk, and then assessed artificially against ideal standards.

To my inexperienced ears, this approach appeared to guide most of the teaching such that we were taught about disorder or impairment rather than differences or diversity, and about cognitive neurological models, anatomy, and physiology to understand clinical presentations. This did not sit easily with my ontological perspective (i.e., view of how the world existed), or the disjunct with the oft cited Royal College of Speech and Language Therapist (RCSLT) premise that speech and language therapy was principally guided by a social model. The commitment to this principle was succinctly demonstrated by their use of the acronym SLCN (Speech, Language and Communication needs) to focus on communicative competence, in contrast to SLI (Speech and Language Impairment) which focuses on linguistic competence, including physical and psychological aetiologies but not social. For me, the elevation of the social model seemed especially prevalent in adult learning disability literature where the policy focus was on providing meaningful interventions that were functionally relevant to the client to improve social participation (Baker et al., 2010).

Clinical guidelines frequently paid heed to the importance of therapists taking account of the environment in their assessments, for example, the extent to which the school, home, or hospital supported alternative and augmentative forms of communication to plan an intervention (RCSLT, 2016). Money (1997), and later Money and Thurman's (2002) "Means, Reasons, and Opportunities" model had a strong influence over how therapists viewed the assessment and management of the referred individual. It alerted them to (what the authors called) *real-world understanding* or situational understanding: the need to think not only about the person's means of communication (if they used speech, signing, visual supports, objects, or so on), but also their reasons and opportunities to communicate, and the ways environments influenced clients' understanding. Without reasons or opportunities to communicate, individuals would be unable to demonstrate communication competencies and not able to participate in social activities. Moreover, routines and predictability were central to how clients made sense of their daily lives.

However, while a consideration of the environment is necessary for effective assessments and treatments of communication, it is important to be aware that this is not the whole story in terms of addressing the implications of the social narrative. I shall show in this chapter how language-based analytic approaches, specifically CA and DA, in research have shone a spotlight on how communication is not just the sum of the individuals language production but is also the product of the actual interaction itself. My unease with the overly dominant individualized and medicalized approach in speech and language therapy was that for me talk is a social constructed as well as an anatomical, physiological, and neurological phenomenon. It is not just social because we talk to other people, but it is social because the medium in which we talk (language) is socially constructed and meaning making (via language) is also socially constructed. The content and the shape of our conversations happen because of the interaction between people not just because of individuals wishing to relay certain messages. This theoretical positioning underpins my ensuing clinical practice in learning disability and mental health services, and later my interest in discourse approaches in my PhD.

The UNITE PhD research study

In the summer of 2017, the National Institute for Health Research (NIHR) awarded me a PhD studentship to study staff and autistic patient communication in psychiatric hospital ward rounds. This study is called UNITE (Staff and Autistic Communication in Mental Health Hospital Ward Rounds), and it was given full approval by the Health Research Authority in March 2019.

Prior to the award, I had been working as a therapist in acute and rehabilitation psychiatric services providing communication and dysphagia support to hospitalized patients. I noticed that many of the referrals to speech and language therapy were for autistic individuals diagnosed with additional mental health concerns, such as depression, psychosis, and personality disorder, as well as challenging behaviour. Often, it was their behaviour that challenged that triggered the referral, either because of observed expressive and receptive communication difficulties, sensory issues, staff inability to engage patients or patients isolating themselves. My interest in ward rounds grew because while they were perceived by patients as difficult meetings to navigate, I was aware that ward rounds were earmarked as the primary space for teams to share clinical information and involve the patient in care decisions.

Ward rounds are interaction encounters where multi-disciplinary teams, patients, and their families come together to review patient care. For this reason, they could be viewed as critical sites to demonstrate effective communication practices including the use of reasonable adjustments as well as other involvement strategies. My research question was formulated out of this *clinical noticing*, from first-hand experience on the wards of autistic patients' difficulties with hospital communication practices especially patient ward rounds. It was also influenced by the literature and the clear absence of research about autistic adult experiences in hospital, lack of qualitative studies of ward rounds, and limited studies on the clinical use of reasonable adjustments in practice.

The wider rationale for the research question is that it addresses health policy concerns about poor communication between services and staff teams, minimal involvement of vulnerable hospitalized patients in decision-making and the call for reasonable adjustments to ensure appropriate care for people with communication impairments (Royal College of Speech and Language Therapists, 2013). The question of how to prevent poor patient treatment and even death in NHS hospitals and public care homes, and the ensuing scandals in learning disability and autistic services, has focussed in large part on the issue of communication (Department of Health, 2012). This policy context, and the resulting governmental rhetoric regarding a demand for person-centred care, gives a framework for understanding why a study on patient-staff communication in hospital ward rounds is vital.

When I started on my PhD journey, despite many years in higher education, I had never heard of conversational analysis, or other discourse approaches like discursive psychology, nor was I aware of the concept of naturalistic data. I had not considered how real-world research linked directly to health improvement via practice-based evidence. My clinical training had elevated the status of evidence-based practice where research informed frontline activity, but it had neglected to identify how naturalistic studies of clinical or practice-based activity could generate evidence (O'Reilly and Kiyimba, 2015). The aim of this chapter is to give readers an idea of why I think these methodologies bring something to the clinician's table. They are not musty academic debates; they are relevant and useful for practitioners and I shall outline why.

As we have seen, my own academic background as a sociologist, and clinical background in adult learning disability and mental health as an SLT already oriented me to an approach to my work broadly aligned to the social model of disability (Oliver, 1983). This model views social organisation not individual deficiencies as causing disability, including communication disabilities. With its roots in a Marxist approach, it views capitalist socio-political organization as creating disability because of its need to identify active working age adults to generate capital for the economy. According to writers like Finkelstein, the disability discourse gained cultural currency because of a capitalist doctrine that required a way to distinguish between productive and the non-productive adults (Finkelstein, 1981). The social model's origin as a critical perspective on how disability was perceived has been somewhat lost in the populist adoption of the model by professional bodies such as the RCSLT. It was also never intended as a theory to explain the experiences of all disabled people (Oliver, 2013).

Originally, the idea of the *social model* evolved to understand the needs of males with physical disabilities, such as those that resulted from war-time injuries. Their disabilities were explained as society-made because proper access was not available to those in wheelchairs. Yet, the model's translation to communication disabilities is not as simple. If someone is autistic and has difficulties expressing themselves in social situations, it is not as easy to find an environmental wrongdoer. What it can do is shine a light on the importance of indirect interventions aimed at modifying how communication partners interact with impaired individuals.

Many well-respected adult intervention packages aim to support communication partners to make changes in how they talk to their partners (Lock et al., 2010). These types of approaches work from the premise that change needs to occur in how others communicate rather than expecting the effected individual to modify their communication. The rationale for this approach with autistic adults is that their condition is agreed to be largely fixed because it is neuro-developmental, associated with impairment in the brain and present from birth. Thus, there is room for change to be facilitated in how others communicate with them and addressing change in staff, family, and friends. This clinical starting point, where indirect approaches are conceptualized as more appropriate than direct approaches, has a strong tradition in SLT practice. It is interesting to note that the rationale for the indirect approach sits alongside a biological perspective on the aetiology of autism.

Significantly, for the messages from this chapter, this indirect approach also has a close affinity with the methodological approach taken in the PhD. It also aligns with conversation analytic and discourse approaches that view talk as constructed in interactions.

CA-inspired discourse approaches in UNITE

I have explained the rationale for the research topic, and now I shall outline the discourse approach in the methodology and the reasons for this decision. The UNITE study started with an interest in *the experiences* of staff and families of ward rounds and *the work* they do to support autistic communication and patient involvement with a focus on communication improvement. I fixed on the idea of conducting qualitative reflexive interviews to facilitate collaborative discussions with patient and staff about their experiences and to utilise my skills as a practitioner. I was also interested in exploiting the clinical-academic perspective that I brought to the research and exploring this dual role in the research (see also Hart and Eccles, this volume for a discussion of dual roles). In short, I started with an interest essentially in *what people say* about their experiences (their remembered experiences) as I was not aware of other methods to examine these questions.

However, my *methodological turn* took shape as I started reading the academic literature, and I discovered conversation analysis, video-based research, as well as ideas about *natural* methods and *atypical* communication. This shifted my thinking about how meaningful it is to ask people about their remembered experiences and re-orientated my research design towards looking at what happens in real talk. In short, my interest refocussed on *communication as performed* as opposed to *communication as imagined*.

These academic debates resonated with my clinical practice. Due to my strongly held view that therapy had to be meaningful to clients and functional, I had a keen interest in understanding how autistic individuals communicated *in real life*. The academic literature in this area provided critical learning points for clinical practice and a marriage was born. The critical points of overlap between clinical practice and the academic focus in CA were: its social approach to language, emphasis on real talk, focus on interaction, and a view of impairment as being *additionally* socially (re) produced within interaction. These overlaps are examined in more detail below when I address the value of CA and DA to speech and language practice.

I have detailed the journey of my interest in the approach, now I shall turn to a closer look at what conversation analysis is and why it is useful for SLTs. Conversation analysis has its roots in several disciplines including linguistics and social psychology, but it is commonly accepted to be influenced mostly by sociology. Its founding father, Harvey Sacks, was a sociologist, and together with Emmanuel Schegloff and Gail Jefferson, they provided a detailed account of the approach that gave theoretical and practical direction for the emergence of the methodology (Sacks, 1992) for a posthumously published series of Sack's lectures). CA was strongly shaped by Garfinkel's work on ethnomethodology with its central concern with how people mutually construct social order in their everyday routines and practices (Garfinkel, 1984), Goffman's scholarship on the "interaction order" (Goffman, 1983), and the tradition of phenomenology (Moran, 2000).

CA positioned itself within key theoretical debates in the social sciences, especially sociology. It took a perspective on the thorny sociological question about the nature of the relationship between agency (individual level) and structure (society level), stating that a focus on participant concerns in interactions could identify how structural issues are made relevant in everyday encounters, if at all. CA could also shed light on how people achieve inter-subjectivity, i.e., how we share a common understanding of society and each other's actions as this could also be studied by close analysis of talk sequences in interactions.

CA became an ally to scholars working in clinical linguistics who also viewed disordered communication as "rule-governed" despite the presence of an impairment, and that by shedding light on the rules and organisation, light could also be shed on the disorder itself (Perkins and Howard, 1995). This position was in sharp contrast to Noam Chomsky's position that all performed talk is chaotic and not orderly. Despite ontological, epistemological and theoretical differences between CA and clinical linguistics, due in large part to the latter's reductionist view of language, a joint concern with how local context shapes talk output and a view of talk as inherently orderly even when it is atypical provided points of mutual enquiry for both traditions (see Body and Muskett (2013) for a discussion of the application of CA to clinical linguistics, and the tension caused by different lineage).

CA also positioned itself in relation to social psychology. Together with discursive psychologists (another strand of DA), scholars challenged the dominant paradigm of cognitivism in social psychology in the 1980s and influenced a transformation in the discipline (Edwards and Potter, 1992). They proposed that so-called "psychological" phenomena like memory, attitudes and identity were socially constructed rather than individualized, internalized, and cognitivist entities.

This foregrounding of the emerging discipline of CA provided a boundaried focus for its form of enquiry as: "the study of recorded, naturally occurring talk in interaction" (Hutchby and Wooffitt, 2008, p. 12). In this quote, the authors highlight two central features of conversation analysis. The first is a concern with naturally occurring data, that is data that would exist regardless of the research not data that is researcher generated, such as interviews and focus group (Kiyimba, Lester, and O'Reilly, 2019). It is video or audio recorded data, so that analysis focusses on real-life sequences of turns rather than reported versions of what happens.

Secondly, CA is interested in *talk in interaction* rather than language per se, that is, "the interactional organisation of social activities" (Hutchby and Wooffitt, 2008, p. 12). Words are viewed as objects or products of activities rather than purely atomized and semantic units of study. CA is about the rough and tumble of authentic interaction, and this includes not just the verbal conversation but the vocalizations and non-verbal elements too, such as, laughter, eye gaze, and proxemics. There is a growing body of research on multi-modal communication that captures the interactional work of these paralinguistic features (Streeck, Goodwin, and Le Baron, 2011).

Significantly, CA research has provided new ways to conceptualize the communication of autistic adults; not as flawed, deficient or impaired but as competent and co-constructed in interactions with conversational partners. In highlighting the *interactional* character of talk, it has positioned autistic people as co-constructors with their conversational partners and questioned the individualized notions of impairment at the heart of medicalized discourses. The CA community talk about *atypical communication* rather than disordered or impaired communication, thereby locating the autistic person's communication within more of a social-constructionist approach instead of a medical one.

In so doing, CA can be harnessed to challenge the medical model's reliance on normal/abnormal thresholds in diagnosing autism and the presumption that a diagnosis means abnormal communication. By re-labelling communication as atypical it circumvents the needs to position communication as abnormal with its moral connotations and sees it instead as different perhaps, but not wrong, and certainly not inhuman as the term abnormal could suggest. It also challenges researchers to think more carefully about the how thresholds are driven by neuro-typical definitions of normality.

This re-conceptualization has reinvigorated the need to consider the *local context* in which interactions have taken place, and to recognise the role of the conversation partner in the communication. This means that there is greater scope for acknowledging that changes in how staff communicate may improve the performance of autistic communicators. It can also provide a rationale for explaining why autistic individuals may perform better in some contexts than others, for example, at home rather than at work or school (Musket, 2017, in O'Reilly, Lester and Muskett, 2017). Ultimately, it leaves open the possibility that staff making reasonable adjustments will lead to increased opportunities for patient involvement.

The value of CA, DA, and natural data for SLTs

Speech and language therapy intervention is often aimed at significant others in the lives of the impaired individual. For example, SPPARC is aimed at the carers and partners of people who have had a stroke and have a resulting aphasia condition, and the Hanen Parent Child Interaction Programme focusses on the families of children with speech and language impairments (Eyberg, 1988). It is typical in speech and language therapy practice for recommendations and training to be indirect, that is, aimed at communication partners rather than the impaired person. The premise of popular interventions like Communication Passports is that change needs to occur in how others communicate with the person rather than insistence on changes from the affected individual, and their use highlights the need for communication partners to make reasonable adjustments, rather than the onus being on the individual client (Millar and Caldwell, 1997). It is interesting that such a widely used and key tool in therapists' interventions box has such a poor evidence base; it is just the kind of intervention that language-based approaches could examine how and why they work.

The value of a CA-like discourse analytic approach for speech and language therapy practice is three-fold and derives from: its methodological toolkit, a body of empirical work especially in the field of atypical interaction, and a focus on natural data. A caveat is needed here; I can only give a flavour of what the added benefits of these approaches are for the practitioner in these three areas as this is a personal and short piece. Suffice to say that there are many excellent introductory books on these approaches if practitioners have their taste buds wetted. For example, Stokoe (2019) has written a book aimed at the general public, entitled *Talk: The Science of Talk*, and two others books of interest for practitioners are an introductory text on applied CA (Lester and O'Reilly, 2018) and the other on naturally occurring data (Kiyimba et al., 2019).

A methodological toolkit to identify communication concerns

In terms of the value of the approaches, the first point to note is that CA-inspired discourse approaches provide an *over-flowing bag of tools* consisting of concepts, devices and resources for the clinician to examine language. The tools are not just familiar linguistic concepts, such as word classes or syntax, but *interactional* elements, such as repair (other and self-initiated), adjacency pairs, preferred responses, turn constructional units, hedging, back channelling, and so on, in the case of CA. I say over-flowing as I know from many conversations with people over the course of my research that they often report that they find CA to be impenetrable, too focussed on the tiniest detail in talk and too jargonistic. The last criticism is levelled as especially ironic by critics who compare the stated aim of CA to provide a participant voice against the highly professionalized and abstract terminology.

In response, I have learnt that the toolkit is large but that practitioners can take parts of it and use it flexibly. This may be heresy to purer CA theorists, but I feel adaptation is legitimate when it is done with the goal of improving clinical care. The terminology is complex and there is clinician learning involved, but the jargon is for clinicians or researcher to use to understand the communication at hand: it is not intended to be the language used for participant feedback. CA also comes with a strong emphasis on a form of detailed transcription named after Jefferson which does take time to learn and practice. This transcription details words, pauses, intonation, volume, overlapping speech, vocalizations, and even laughter. However, there are lighter versions available for the busy clinician and their use will still constitute an improvement on a simpler orthographic or phonetic transcription, albeit not the CA gold standard. Many dedicated speech and language therapists are already trained in phonetic transcription, have a good ear for auditory nuances, and they will understand the rationale for a more detailed transcription even though they may have to learn a different approach in the Jeffersonian method.

The beauty of a CA approach is that it provides a rich methodology about how to analyse real talk. It is a nuts-and-bolts toolkit for examining real conversations. The value for the therapist is that they can see in detail from the data and the sequences of turn-taking how the participants shaped (and were influenced) by the talk *as it occurred*. This means that the therapist can see where there were *problems* in the talk (identified due to the negative consequences for the client rather than clinician-led ideas about what constitutes a problem). It also helps the therapist to see what kinds of turns worked well for the client and which did not. The therapist will be able to see from the data how the participants responded to different types of approaches and what ensued (did the opener close the patient down, did the pause result in participant continuing their turn or not, and so on). For example, research investigating how rapport is generated between therapists and clients in adult mental health forensic settings by Dobbinson (2016; and this volume) details her experiences of working therapeutically with a learning disabled autistic male using a CA approach.

In relation to my own research, this close examination of talk means that ways of interacting in the hospital ward round that were hitherto un-noticed are laid bare. It is not so much about the content of what is said but *how* things are done; the routines, processes, language and rhetoric that reveal how staff manage care work through their interactions.

A long history of empirical research on atypical communication

The second value derives from the empirical findings of CA and DA studies and their application to both assessment and management in speech and language therapy. Again, I have to be selective for the purposes of the chapter and so I am focusing on a specific branch of empirical work; a well-established body of work going back to the end of the 1970s on *Atypical Communication,* examining communication where one of the conversational partners has a communication impairment. Wilkinson (2019) has written a very useful article summarizing the impact of CA studies on our understanding of atypical communication, and specifically how different communication impairments manifest in differently diagnosed communication disorders, and what their similarities and differences are in interactional terms. In a sense, this reframes our diagnostic boundaries so that conditions like autism, traumatic brain injury, and dementia are viewed more similarly in interactional terms because they all manifest similar interactional similarities. These conditions are predominantly cognitive impairments and disrupt the performance of social actions. Wilkinson notes that their pragmatic impairment means that, "the inappositeness may be linked to the sequential/topical position of the utterance or its apparent function there, including initiating or developing a topic" (Button and Casey, quoted in Wilkinson, 2019, p. 291). For example, providing information as if it is new or introducing topics that are not relevant.

Other communicative impairments demonstrate their atypicality because they disrupt by delaying the progressivity of the turn as a dysfluency could, or show atypical difficulties with hearing, understandability, and intelligibility, for example, as found in a hearing impairment, an intellectual disability or aphasia. These distinctions highlight the importance of the polarised concepts of competency versus performance that should also be elevated in speech and language therapy practice. Wilkinson (2019) finds that autistic individuals are not incompetent as such in relation to their social communication; instead they are impaired performers.

For the novice, Wilkinson (2019) gives a useful potted history of the development of CA work on atypical interaction. He highlights the work of academics examining a wide variety of communication disorders, for example, dysfluency, aphasia, dementia, autism, mental health, learning disability, and traumatic head injury, that could be applied to SLT work. He highlights that the research emphasis has been on acquired disorders not developmental disorders. There is some CA research in speech therapy on aphasia and children's speech interventions but markedly less on autistic adults and in mental health. Despite this growing community of SLT researchers working in CA and DA, there is not a lot of awareness among the SLT profession generally about these methodologies, and this may be due to an over-emphasis on pre-registration programmes on medical approaches.

This CA work also has implications for clinical assessments. Researchers have investigated therapists' interactions with clients using CA approaches, for example in areas such as child autism (Local and Wootton, 1995) and aphasia (Wilkinson, 2014). Maynard and Turowetz (2017) analysed the process of autism assessments and evidenced how children demonstrate desired communication competencies that are un-accounted for by clinicians. Using video-recordings of real-life assessments, they show how children's performance of social communication skills goes unnoticed by the assessor because the performance was outside of the formal sequence of the assessment or demonstrated in a different way. For example, one child was not able to do the demonstration task at the allotted time to show social imagination and non-verbal communication skills, but she did at a later point, show both these skill sets when she pretended to take tissues and sneeze; *a pretend showing* rather than a pretend telling (Maynard and Turowetz, 2017).

Others have conducted studies examining how the therapist changes their conversational turns to anticipate the communication impairments of their clients, thereby reifying and maintaining the atypicality of the interactions. For example, planned repair work of client "mistakes" with sound production in dysarthria (Wilkinson, 2013) or vocabulary in aphasic speech (Wilkinson, Beeke, and Maxim, 2003), alters the natural give and take of the conversation so that atypicality is reproduced. The lesson for the therapist is to be aware that their interactions are also changing the interaction dynamic and be mindful that pedagogic goals (to learn how to say X) establish power hierarchies within the client–therapist relationship.

The value of conceptualizing and utilizing natural data

This highlights the third feature of value of CA-inspired approaches, namely the focus on *natural data*. In the case highlighted above, videoing captured the child's performance because it could show in real time how the child used *multimodal communication* interactionally, and how this was critical to understand autistic communication, i.e., the non-verbal aspects of the interaction including gesture, facial expression, body language, and proxemics. There is clearly some benefit to video-recording some or parts of clinical sessions or everyday interactions of the participant. A careful watching and re-playing of client interactions can potentially open up not just new ways of understanding the client's communication but support a more holistic view of the person competencies. Interestingly, there are signs that there is support among SLTs for some of the key ideas of CA regarding the role of naturalistic data. Last year, there was a paper presented to the RCSLT conference on the benefits of naturalistic sampling. The finding was that a naturalistic language sample elicits more competencies than structured assessments (Bates and Stewart, 2019). In order to obtain this, therapists need to be audio-recording or videoing as part of their routine work, and addressing ethical considerations as part of this, especially consent.

Anecdotally, it seems a lot of speech and language therapists in practice unknowingly focus on expressive language as a set of individual skills that are inherent to the individual. This practice may be unwittingly encouraged because of formal speech and language assessments that sustain the idea that skills live within the person and are measurable objectively. In sharp contrast to this way of working, CA fosters a re-framing of communication as interactionally constructed. Muskett, Body, and Perkins (2013) showed how even in the delivery of a simple semantic assessment, the types of turns taken by the therapist influenced the child's turns. Even simple back-channelling turns by the therapist where the therapist says "um" to encourage response, or where they paused or used longer silences, changed the shape of what the child demonstrated or not. In short, CA prompts therapists to think about the interaction and their role within it, and not just to focus on the client's responses.

Box 12.1 below summarizes three practical tips for improving communication arising out of a CA inspired approach to clinical practice.

Personal reflections: Videoing, reflexive interviews and improving practice

When I embarked on the PhD, I was not aware of the training that would be involved. I was also not mindful about what being a clinical-academic was, nor how this dual role would influence the research. I had undertaken a couple of academic courses whilst working as an SLT but in the main I was solely clinical. As a clinician, I barely found time to visit the on-site library to access literature or to identify articles to support my practice, despite the demands from clinical leaders to evidence our work. I felt that my literature search skills were poor, and I was not providing robust rationales for my practice.

On the adult in-patient mental health wards, I noticed that the speech and language therapy team were getting many referrals for autistic individuals. They were referred because staff did not know how best to communicate with clients, and they were perceived to be a problem in some way. For example, refusing to come out of their bedrooms, not participating in social activities or being demanding of staff time (repetitively asking for leave, cigarettes, and so on). Staff would also refer for an assessment of receptive communication or mental capacity assessments.

Box 12.1   Practical tips
Practical tips for improving communication

- Gather data that is *as natural as possible* to work with real interactions rather than imagined or artificial interactions. This may mean recording parts of clinical sessions or the client interacting with people as part of their normal routines.
- Look at the data *as an interaction* rather than as the product of separate entities talking. Focus on the ways in which the conversation unfolds and the kinds of inputs of all the speakers (including clinician) not only the impaired individual.
- Consider how the client may be using non-verbal communication to indicate a *social action*. For example, shorter-than-expected responses may not be indicative of an inability to construct a syntactically fuller response but a resistance. Look at how you as a therapist may be influencing the responses available to the client.

My attendance at the person's ward rounds was a necessary part of working with the autistic individual in hospital, to ensure my work integrated with the wider team approach. It was important that the speech therapy input was part of a broader team approach so that there were shared objectives among the staffing group. I quickly became aware that ward rounds were difficult places for autistic in-patients, and that anecdotally there was an over-reliance on verbal communication and an absence of any reasonable adjustments in the form of alternative or augmentative communication methods (AAC). My initial impression was that ward rounds often did more harm than good: they were stressful for people and (in some cases) led to behaviours that were subsequently challenging for services. I saw first-hand patients anxiously pacing up and down corridors or head banging prior to ward rounds especially if they were later than scheduled, and patients becoming aggressive and or non-communicative following a meeting because of their feelings or events during the meetings.

As a SLT, I knew that autistic people often found talking difficult, especially in groups and with people with whom they are not familiar. A cursory search for any literature on this area turned up very little of any direct help or relevance. Some ward studies were available, but these were mainly survey-based and there were some articles examining how staff over-estimated the communication skills of clients with learning disabilities and autism. I was mindful of the need to be an evidenced-based practitioner and this drive, coupled with the desire to improve practice, influenced my decision to apply for an NIHR research award to examine how care work is done in ward rounds in staff interactions with this patient group.

I was keen that my research adopt an approach towards my patients that conceptualized their impairment and communication as being socially constructed, and that it exploit my role as a clinician to facilitate reflective discussions with staff to improve communication practices as an action-oriented aspect of the project. Conversation analysis and other discourse approaches it inspired, provided a methodological toolkit to examine staff and patient talk as well as a theoretical orientation about talk as performance.

There were significant challenges getting the research off the ground. Obtaining ethical approval proved tricky and it took over a year to get the green light. Hospital managers had reservations about the value of videoing due to concerns about potentially observing poor practices and the desire to maintain professional reputations. Concerns regarding the so-called "vulnerability" of patients were also a major sticking point in my ethics application. I addressed fears about patient coercion by detailing in writing processes to safeguard research participants and protections. Some were also sceptical about the "naturalness" of videoing, stating that I would see staff on their best behaviour and not as they would usually work. About this, I could cite evidence that the presence of a camera may alter natural conversation for a very short time initially, but that participants forgot about the camera and would interact with one another normally. The ethics approval also stipulated that I needed to obtain all the consents of the participants' consents prior to any video-recording. Interestingly, it was not difficult to get patient consent; the problem was getting all the staff consents in advance of the scheduled meeting. I quickly learnt to ask a key informant which staff were expected to be at the meeting, and then to ensure that I had spoken to everyone that I could before the ward round took place to lessen any chance of a staff member objecting.

The transcribed video-recordings detail the inter-group exchanges and provide a closer representation of what goes on in the ward round meetings rather than relying on people's memory. From these data, I can examine *what* is talked about (topics), *how* phenomena are talked about, and the ward round *processes*. Each ward round is followed up with three audio-recorded interviews; a patient interview conducted first followed by two staff interviews. The interviews provide an opportunity for me to explore participants' experiences of communication, ward rounds, and hospital. I can use my skills and knowledge as a speech therapist to support a reflective interview to think about what communication approaches work and why. Whilst this improvement activity is done in the moment (during the interviews), I also intend to use the research output to support practitioners to communicate better with autistic individuals in hospital. After I have completed the analysis of both video and interview data sets, I will be able to use the more detailed findings (in a summative way) to develop communication training and/or guidelines for staff. In this way, I can support communication improvement as the research evolves and as an endpoint. By doing this research, I want to generate some of that much-needed evidence that I mentioned at the start of this reflection, and to have contributed to a strong body of work on atypical communication with an added *group setting* dynamic.

Conclusion: Communication as performance

The chapter has given a flavour of my academic learning grappling with language-focussed methodologies, and how I believe this learning can shine a spotlight on developing new ways to work in speech and language therapy. I have summarized the value of marrying practice with CA and CA-inspired discourse approaches like discursive psychology. First, the methodological value in the metaphor of the toolkit. Secondly, the empirical value, in relation to a strong body of work on atypical communication, and lastly, in relation to our need to exploit our use of natural data, not least because it has empirical validity for evidence-based work. Fasulo and Sterponi (2016) powerfully argue that CA does not reject the idea of neurological aetiology, only the dominance of the deficit model and significantly; CA re-focusses attention onto competencies and interaction. My interest is how we can adopt more CA-like methodologies in practice and shine a spotlight on communication as a social performance. Communication can then be viewed not just as the sum of two individual performers, but instead as the unique product of the interaction performance itself.

References

Baker, V. et al., 2010. *Adults with Learning Disabilities (ALD)*. RCSLT, London.

Bates, S., Stewart, J., 2019. "The joy of syntax": What we can learn from two different sampling contexts. Paper presented to the RCSLT 2019 Conference.

Body, R., Muskett, T., 2013. The case for multi-modal analysis of atypical interaction: Questions, answers and gaze in play involving a child with autism. *Clinical Linguistics and Phonetics* 27 (10–11), 837–850.

Brechin, A., Liddiard, P., Swain, J. (Eds.), 1981. *Handicap in a Social World: A Reader*. Hodder Arnold, London.

Department of Health, 2012. *Transforming Care: A National Response to Winterbourne View Hospital*. Department of Health, London.

Dobbinson, S., 2016. Conversation with an adult with features of autism spectrum disorder in secure forensic care. In: O'Reilly, M., Lester, J. (Eds.), *The Palgrave Handbook of Adult Mental Health*. Palgrave MacMillan, Basingstoke.

Edwards, D., Potter, J., 1992. *Discursive Psychology*. SAGE, London.

Eyberg, S., 1988. Parent-child interaction therapy. *Child and Family Behaviour Therapy* 10, 33–46.

Fasulo, A., Sterponi, L., 2016. Understanding children's mental health conditions in their interactional environment: Conversational analysis and autism. *TPM* 23 (4), 453–470.

Finkelstein, V., 1981. Disability and the Helper/Helped Relationship. An Historical View. In: Brechin, A., Liddiard, P., Swain, J. (Eds.), *Handicap in a Social World*. Hodder Arnold.

Garfinkel, H., 1984. *Studies in Ethnomethodology*. Polity Press, Cambridge.

Goffman, E., 1983. The interaction order. *American Sociological Review* 48, 1–17.

Hutchby, I., Wooffitt, R., 2008. *Conversation Analysis*. Polity, Cambridge.

Kiyimba, N., Lester, N., O'Reilly, M., 2019. *Using Naturally Occurring Data in Qualitative Health Research: A Practical Guide*. Springer, Cham, Switzerland.

Lester, N., O'Reilly, M., 2018. *Applied Conversational Analysis*. SAGE, Thousand Oaks, CA.

Local, J., Wootton, T., 1995. Interactional and phonetic aspects of immediate echolalia in autism: A case study. *Clinical Linguistics and Phonetics* 9 (2), 155–184.

Lock, S., Wilkinson, R., Bryan, K., Maxim, J., Edmundson, A., Bruce, C.arolyn, Moir, D., 2010. Supporting partners of people with aphasia in relationships and conversation (SPPARC). *Int. J. Lang. Commun. Disord.* 36, 25–30.

Maynard, D., Turowetz, J., 2017. Doing diagnosis: Autism, interaction order, and the use of narrative in clinical talk. *Social Psychology Quarterly* 80 (3), 254–275.

Millar, S., Caldwell, M., 1997. Personal communication passports. Paper presented at the SENSE Conference, Westpark Centre, University of Dundee, Scotland (13 September 1997).

Money, D., 1997. A comparison of three approaches to delivering a speech and language therapy service to people with learning disabilities. *European Journal of Disorders of Communication 32 (4), 449–466*.

Money, D., Thurman, S., 2002. *Means, reasons and opportunities model for communication. Speech and Language Therapy in Practice,* Winter Issue, 4–6.

Moran, D., 2000. *Introduction to Phenomenology.* Routledge, London.

Muskett, T., Body, R., Perkins, M., 2013. A discursive psychology critique of semantic verbal fluency assessment and its interpretation. *Theory and Psychology* 23 (2), 205–226.

Musket, T., 2017. Using conversation analysis to assess the language and communication of people on the autism spectrum: a case-based tutorial. In: O'Reilly, M., Lester, N.L., Muskett, T. (Eds.), *A Practical Guide to Social Interaction Research in Autism Spectrum Sisorders.* Palgrave MacMillan, London.

Oliver, M., 1983. *Social work with disabled people.* Macmillan, Basingstoke.

Oliver, M., 2013. The social model: 30 years on. *Disability and Society* 28 (7), 1024–1026.

O'Reilly, M., Kiyimba, N., 2015. *Advanced Qualitative Research.* SAGE, London.

Perkins, M., Howard, S., 1995. *Case Studies in Clinical Linguistics.* Whurr, London.

Royal College of Speech and Language Therapists, 2013. *Five Good Communication Standards: Reasonable Adjustments to Communication that Individuals with Learning Disability and/or Autism should expect in Specialist Hospital and Residential Settings.* RCSLT, London.

Royal College of Speech and Language Therapists, 2016. *Inclusive Communication and the Role of Speech and Language Therapist.* RCSLT, London.

Sacks, H., 1992. *Lectures on Conversation (Vols 1 and 2, ed. G.Jefferson).* Blackwell Publishing, Oxford.

Stokoe, E., 2019. *Talk: The Science of Conversation.* Robinson, London.

Streeck, J., Goodwin, C., Le Baron, C. (Eds.), 2011. *Embodied Interaction. Language and Body in the Material World.* Cambridge University Press, Cambridge.

Wiggins, S., 2017. *Discursive Psychology. Theory, Method and Applications.* SAGE, London.

Wilkinson, R., 2013. Conversation analytic investigations of dysarthria and hearing impairment: The impact of motor and sensory impairments in social interaction. *Journal of Interactional Research in Communication Disorders* 4 (1), 1–26.

Wilkinson, R., 2014. Intervening with conversation analysis in speech and language therapy: Improving aphasic conversation. *Research on Language and Social Interaction* 47 (3), 219–238.

Wilkinson, R., 2019. Atypical interaction: Conversation analysis and communicative impairments. *Research on Language and Social Interaction* 52 (3), 281–299.

Wilkinson, R., Beeke, S., Maxim, J., 2003. Adapting to conversations: On the use of linguistic resources by speakers with fluent aphasia in the construction of turns in talk. In: Goodwin, C. (Ed.), *Conversation and Brain Damage.* Oxford University Press, New York, NY, pp. 59–89.

Chapter 13

Developing supra-vision using naturally occurring video material within supervision

Sarah Helps

Introduction

The ultimate purpose of clinical supervision is to ensure that service users receive the best possible and most effective care. The use of Video Conversation Analysis (VCA) within supervision offers practitioners the opportunity to examine recordings of naturally occurring practice so as to critically reflect on and improve their part in the conversational dance of the therapeutic process.

In this chapter, I will firstly describe the importance of supervision, then the process of video review in supervision. Using a detailed example, I will outline how VCA can be used to explore how clinical conversation works, specifically in relation to the contribution of the therapist. I will then conclude by emphasizing the benefits of using VCA to connect micro-examinations of dialogue to broader layers of context. Examples are from systemically informed practice, but my comments on VCA and the process of supra-vision are applicable to clinicians working with any therauptic modality whether in self-, individual, or group supervision.

Supervision is a crucial part of practice

Clinical supervision is a crucial part of clinical practice and is mandated throughout the professional life span. It involves processes of reflection in, on, and for action, and seeks to connect research and theory with practice and organizational governance.

Supervision has multiple aims: it can be used to teach a particular therapeutic approach, for example to trainees learning how to deliver a particular mode of practice, or it can be to provide space in which to reflect on one's therapeutic practice (Fruggeri, 2018). Different supervisory purposes call for different areas of focus. Fruggeri suggests that if the focus is primarily on skills training then the object of examination is the practice of the therapist. But if the focus is reflection, then it is what goes on between therapist and client that is key. Of course, as the client is not present in the supervision setting, the focus is on the story or sense that the therapist makes of this interaction. Other forms of information would be necessary to understand the experience of the client.

In this chapter, I will focus on how VCA enables what might be called supravision, a process whereby the therapist takes up a meta position of looking at themselves and their clients, and at the conversational to-and-fro between therapist and clients that builds meaningful dialogue and that leads to change.

Supervision can take a variety of forms. It might involve live supervision where the supervisor is present during the moment of the work and observes that work either in the room or behind a one-way screen. It might involve self-supervision, where the clinician takes time to review and critically reflect on their work. It might involve meeting as a peer group and engaging in reflexive discussions, or it might involve more hierarchical conversations between a supervisor and a supervisee. Whatever the form of supervision, clear contracting for and clarification of the overall task, including the way that power, accountability, and responsibility play out in the relationship needs to be negotiated.

Most usually, supervision involves retrospective review of practice based on the memory and clinical notes made by the supervisee. Descriptions of practice are created in the relational supervisory context. Therefore, the account of the practice presented during supervision might be far from what "actually" happened. This does not imply any aim or desire on the part of the practitioner or the supervisor to wilfully mislead or fabricate, but merely acknowledges the complex process of memory, recall and communication. Using recordings of clinical work offers an evidence-based alternative to this reliance on the supervisee's memory and note-taking, so enabling the supervisory conversation to start from a basis of what actually happened, rather than on what the clinician recalled happening. Thus, starting supervisory conversations with an examination of actual practice is more reliable, less biased, and therefore likely more effective. While examining recordings of clinical work in supervision has been recommended over decades (Chodoff, 1972), and is highly regarded (Scaife, 2009), there is still little guidance on how to do this.

Using naturally occurring material to learn from and improve clinical practice

Family therapists and other systemically informed clinicians have used recordings to review their work, to explore and develop hypotheses about family communication, and about communication between both therapists and families for decades (McQuown, 1971, Erickson, 2011). Examination of recordings of naturally occurring practice has contributed greatly to basic understandings of communication, including what happens when diverse messages are contained in the verbal and the non-verbal communication (Chapter 3; Dallos and Draper, 2010; O'Reilly and Parker, 2013).

Applied CA is particularly illuminating in studying the detail of what happens in a range of forms of therapeutic interventions and psychotherapy (see Antaki and Wilkinson, 2013; Peräkylä, 2011; Peräkylä, 2011). It has been increasingly used in process research in the systemic psychotherapy field (e.g., Rober, von Eesbeek, and Elliot, 2006; Watson, 2018).

Applied CA has been used as a tool to explore practice by family and systemic psychotherapists over decades (Kramer and Reitz, 1980). Indeed, nearly 30 years ago, Gale and Newfield commented: "Conducting micro-analytical studies of brief interactions between the student-therapist and client(s) can help the student-therapist learn how to use his/her communications (both verbal and non-verbal) effectively…Clinicians need to learn how important their own actions and communications (including micro elements of communication) can be within the therapy session" (p. 163).

Communication with words and bodies

It generally accepted that verbal communication accounts for a small percentage our total communication (Mehrabian, 1972). Whatever the actual percentage, much of communication between people is via bodies not words. We must learn to "read" words in their saying and in their bodied performance in order to understand their meaning. This reading of each other is a particularly important part of the process of getting in tune with each other in the clinic space. For example, there are many ways in which I could ask you how you are. In momentarily planning your response, you might take account of my tone of voice, the way in which I speak the words, my body posture, the movements that accompany my words. We will both make all kinds of assumptions about each other that we will be more or less aware of in our conscious thought. The way in which we read each other is a unique function of what we bring to the situation as individuals and in-the-moment experiences (Helps, 2019). The "embodied turn" in clinical practice and supervision thus encourages us to move beyond a languaged, cognitive practice, to make use of what we see and feel in our bodies as we interact (Nevile, 2015, Bownas and Fredman, 2016, Barbetta and Telfner, 2020).

It is therefore apparent that we cannot just examine the words spoken in the therapeutic encounter, and that our understanding of therapeutic interaction has to involve both words and bodies. As technology has become more portable and as videoing our everyday activities has become a socially normative activity, so the use of video-recording technologies in the clinic room has also become more straightforward.

VCA: Time-consuming but worth it

As a clinician, I am interested in the micro-processes that build broader interactional patterns. This includes the way in which words in their saying are put together, such as pitch and tone of voice, the processes of turn-taking, turn design and sequential positioning, and the visual aspects of interaction as well as the content of words.

I am also interested in the overall arc of the conversations I have with families, which ultimately aim to address the concerns they have that brought them to the service. These are extended sequences, in CA terms what might be referred to as Big Packages (Jefferson, 1988) rather than the micro-excerpts of communication that are often analyzed in pure CA. These extended sequences involve an entry into an issue, an exit from that particular issue and the structure of the sequence itself (Psathas, 1992) and fit with my aim of exploring how the clinical conversation unfolds.

These bigger, extended packages also help to make meaning of the excerpts within the context of the overall conversation more than a more traditional, smaller CA package might. Applications of CA have also been used to explore even bigger packages involving whole clinical sessions and have identified a broad five-part structure, involving introductions, reasons for attendance, problem presentation, decision-making, and session closure (O'Reilly and Parker, 2013, O'Reilly et al., 2015, Lee, 2018).

The analysis of material using VCA can be a time-consuming process. Basic transcription of a minute of conversation can take about up to an hour to transcribe. Jeffersonian transcription with added transcription of visual material can take much longer. In the pressurized confines of therapeutic work within the UK NHS or social care system, is it worth it? I believe that it is. Careful analysis of small segments of practice can shed light on habits, assumptions, prejudices, and biases of practice which then enable us to practice differently, not only in the context of the specific therapeutic work that we bring to supervision but across our caseloads and in future work.

VCA analysis as an entry point for contextual understanding

Considering the nested situation of talk is vital to make a useful analysis within clinical practice. Each word, gesture, or movement, each thing that I can actually see, happens within the context of an interaction, which happens in the context of a relationship, which happens in the context of an episode of talk. The conversation also has an institutional and cultural context.

The focus of VCA could be said to focus on the "speech-and-action-act" level of the levels of context of Co-ordinated Management of Meaning (Cronen, Chen, and Pearce, 1988). I define the speech act as a communication that includes words, the ways in which those words are spoken, gestures, and movements that encompasses what the body does in an inseparable performance with the words. The layers of context above the speech act influence how it is performed. Likewise, the performance of the speech-act can create an implicative force on the layers above (Pearce 2006).

Each speech act can be seen as a *turn at talk.* Each turn at talk belongs within an *adjacency pair*, that is the turn at talk that goes before or after, and relates to the first turn, depending on the kind of turn that each is. A basic adjacency pair example is a question (the first pair-part) of a question or comment and a response to that question or comment (ten Have 207). Multiple adjacency pairs contribute to the overall interactional episode. The importance of this is that each speech act is *influenced by* and *influences* the flow of the conversational episode.

While all layers of context are equally important and ripe for supervisory discussions, there is benefit in punctuating between layers in order to study one aspect in depth.

So, what happens at the level of the institution affects the supervisor, which affects the therapist, which affects the client or family. Likewise, something the family might do might affect the therapist, which in turn affects the supervisor, and so on. These processes are bidirectional, recursive, and also intra-active.

Using VCA in supervision

Having built an argument for the benefits of using VCA in supervision, it is necessary to have a framework within which it can be used. A framework is therefore offered below.

Using VCA in supervision involves selecting a recording, doing preparatory work on it and taking the recording and the work to supervision. The process of using VCA within supervision can be seen sequentially as described below (Figure 13.1):

1   Prior to supervision, select a piece of recording, either at random or because it shows an interaction you are interested in. This might be something that went well in the clinical conversation, an impasse, a moment when you used a particular therapeutic technique, a moment when there was a lapse or a hesitation in the conversation or a moment when an issue of social difference seemed pertinent. Using basic VCA practices, examine the material.
2   In supervision, discuss what you have noticed about the way that the conversation is constructed on the basis of this initial analysis.
3   Discuss what you have noticed about the communication. Engage with questions the supervisor has about your noticings. Start to weave this into your knowledge of the work and of your clinical practice.
4   Discuss what actually happened and hold in mind how this is similar or different to what you thought had happened. Notice what you notice about your actual practice – what delights and surprises you, what challenges you. Pay attention to what other people notice.

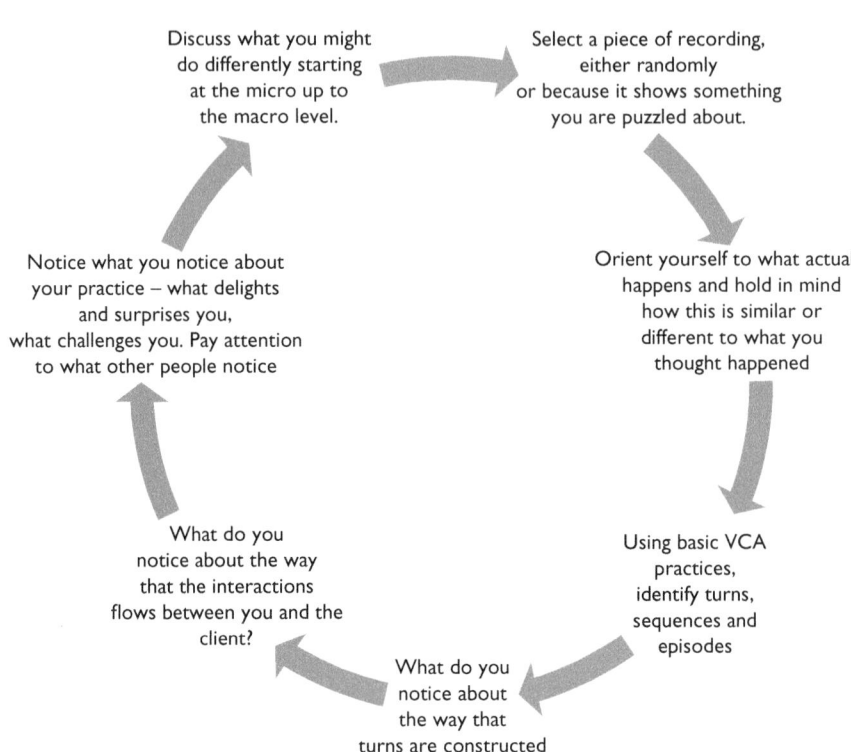

Figure 13.1 The cycle of using VCA within supervision.

5   Discuss what you might do differently based on this analysis.
6   Discuss how your new understandings fit in the broader context of the work.

A worked example: Supervision of Sarah's conversation with Natalie and Bella

I took this episode to peer supervision because the conversation had felt "sticky" and I wondered what I might have missed as the conversation unfolded, and what I might have done differently. A small amount of material is considered below, lasting less than 20 seconds. The rest of the session is not ignored but is held in the background while the initial analysis is undertaken.

This is an excerpt from an initial conversation at a child and family mental health clinic between me, Natalie, aged 14, and Bella.[1] Natalie had been referred to CAMHs for a second opinion because Bella believed there was something "wrong" with Natalie.

Table 13.1 Excerpt 1 supervisory intervention with Natalie and Bella and Sarah

Line	Words	Sarah	Bella	Natalie	Supervisory interventions
11	Me: [Well], maybe you can start off then=I've got all sorts of questions I want to ask you, but maybe you could start off (0.2) and I don't know who's best to start off=just telling me what it is that, that °Natalie's going through°?(3)*	[hand gesture towards both Natalie and Bella] A move to tying up my hair hands quickly settle into my lap	Looking towards me [B makes a small nod]*B looks over at Natalie who continues to stare into her lap	Natalie sits with her eyes down in her lap, hands folded in her lap	What was the intention with the hand gesture to both in the context of inviting them both to start talking? How else might you have invited the family to start to talk about the reasons for coming to CAMHs? What's the ensuing silence about?
12	Bella: Do you want to↑?(6)	Looking towards both of them	B turns to N, speaks and looks at her, makes a brief nervous-laughter like sound	Natalie does not engage at all, offers no eye contact, stares into her lap	What influenced you to hold the silence for so long? What stories can you tell about your relationship to silence?

Bella is sole parent to Natalie and her younger brother. They are a white British family and are experiencing financial and other stressors. The excerpt contains material that is likely very familiar to all clinicians who conduct initial assessments should be within a mental health setting and shows the complexity of navigating this initial session.

Table 13.1 shows the transcript of the observed words and actions[2] alongside the words and the supervisory interventions.

As I prepared the excerpt for supervision, what is immediately noticeable, and what had not been obvious to me before, is my sometimes repetitive, stumbling, hesitant language, as though I am reaching out somewhat in the dark for the words I use.

I next notice the tone and pacing of my words in relation to those of Bella. Although I used Bella's words "What she's been going through", words that she had used in the prior sequence, I did not simply reflect those words back to her and Natalie, but rather I put my own spin on them. My pace was slightly faster than Bella's. Although I appropriate her words, I adapt them to into my own speaking.

My offer to Natalie and Bella to decide who might start to tell me why they are here, carries an implicit suggestion that either mother or daughter might start the conversation, and that I am not going to choose who should start. I realise as I talk about this with my peer supervisor and we think about Tom Anderson's practice (Anderson, 2013), that this systemically inclined way of talking, of opening space for the family to make decisions might feel odd to them, it might be different to how they expect an "expert" to talk to them. I wonder if their ensuing hesitation might suggest that they have had lots of experiences where they have been offered little choice or voice in how the conversation might go on. I also start to wonder if my question is the first move in the overall arc of the conversation to "troubles talk" (Jefferson, 1988).

As can be seen from the transcript above, I ask the pair to tell me why they are here. There is a long pause, and it is clear that the sequence is becoming problematic. My questions, which have moved from ordinary talk into institutional conversation about the reason for coming, have created trouble. Jefferson (1988) has shown that in ordinary conversation there is tension between talking about the "trouble" and talking about "ordinary" things. This tension is greatly apparent in this extract. Benwell and McCreaddie (2016) demonstrated how ordinary social talk could be problematic in clinical encounters, when it stretches so far as to disrupt the institutional agenda. This excerpt suggests that the shift from "ordinary" talk to the institutional agenda, that is, naming the reason for attending – can also create disruption to the conversational flow.

My invitation to the family to start talking is followed by bodily stillness from Natalie and a lengthy silence, perhaps best described in CA terms as an asynchronous moment when mother and daughter give a dispreferred response. My intervention at line 11, commenting that I have "all sorts of questions" (line 11) that I want to ask, is complex. It establishes me as holding epistemic power in asking the questions and in setting myself as perhaps holding expertise. Bella seems happy with my stance as she nods as I speak, but Natalie does not offer any engagement and from her body language I wonder if she is becoming really uncomfortable.

Bella then makes an intervention at line 12 in which she asks a question of her daughter, but does not receive a response. This results in a 6-second pause. This is a very long period of time with no talk. I then pivot to try to rescue and repair a very uncomfortable moment (Table 13.2).

Using a relational question, I quickly pivot (line 13, figure 5) to a process-oriented question and ask how things "usually work" between mother and daughter in these situations. Bella's non-verbal actions (lines 12 to 14)

Table 13.2 Transcript Excerpt 2 supervisory intervention with Natalie and Bella and Sarah

Line	Words	Sarah	Bella	Natalie	Supervisory intervention
13	Me: Who *usually starts talking in these sorts of situations?	*Small hand movements in my lap, looking towards both of them	Gives barely audible grimace-laugh, continues looking towards N, then moves in her chair, tidying the lay of her shirt	N remains totally still, makes no contact with anyone in the room	What made you go to that question then? What issues of social similarity and difference do you think were influencing this moment of the conversation?
14	R1: Bella: If you ask the questions, maybe *(haha) it'd be () easier.		looks back to me, *shaking her head, grimace-smiling		
15	Me: Yeah. Okay.				

communicate her great discomfort far more powerfully than do her words. Bella gives a small laugh-like sound, shifts in her chair, shakes her head at me, and speaks with what I read to be an embarrassed tone to her voice. I follow Bella's request, in an attempt to end the trouble and to reduce her discomfort, by agreeing with her and then asking her some questions (line 15).

The VCA analysis enables me to tune in at great depth to see what my words and bodied actions **do** to the family, and then to see how they respond to my words. Examining the dialogical process in this close way enables me to hypothesise about what is helpful and what I might do differently in the future.

In presenting this excerpt and in listening to supervisory questions about what influenced me to go this way or that, about what led me to ask that question then, I start to think about power. I can't "know" why I did this or that, my post-hoc explanations are shaped by the supervisory questions posed, and by myriad other things (theory, more practice, research, personal experiences, etc.) that have affected my practice between the clinical session and the supervisory conversation. But in the observation of the material I start to consider much more that I previously had the power of my questions and their perturbation of the family system.

This close analysis helps me understand the power of my questions and how, when the whole of the initial conversation is considered it can take multiple attempts of asking the same question in slightly different ways to construct a rich, shared – if not mutually agreed – description of the reasons for coming to CAMHs (Rober, von Eesbeek, and Elliot 2006).

What difference does a VCA approach make? Evaluating outcomes

Evidencing what direct difference any supervisory process makes to clinical practice is very complex (Bond, 2016; Snowdon, Leggat, and Taylor, 2017; Wilkins et al .2018). However it is widely accepted that developing methods that enable supervisee and supervisor to examine actual rather than retrospectively reported practice presents a more robust opportunity to both safeguard clients and to demonstrate and develop the skills of the clinician (Scaife, 2009; Snowdon et al., 2017).

Creating evidence to show what difference a VCA supervisory practice makes is thus also complicated. Multi-layered longitudinal studies would be needed to track how a certain practice within supervision makes a difference to the work of a therapist or to the families with whom they work. In the absence of these, gathering "conversational evidence" from naturally occurring practice creates processual evidence of how change can be achieved through dialogue between patient and therapist (Strong, Busch, and Couture, 2008).

Conclusions

CA has been successfully used as a means of analysing interventions delivered by a range of health professionals working with a wide range of clinical and non-clinical populations (Antaki and Wilkinson, 2013; Goodwin and Cekaite, 2018). It has proven straightforward to teach clinicians the basics of CA so that they can use it in their everyday work to help their clients improve their communication (Wilkinson, 2014). VCA is a logical next step given the embodied nature of much contemporary mental health practice.

The overarching aim of supervision, whether during training or once a practitioner is qualified, is to develop, maintain, and improve competent practice. Therapy and supervision are collaborative and embodied processes (Bownas and Fredman, 2017). We meet each other with our bodies and our words, and our bodies act as a vehicle through which our words are produced and understood. Our words will "touch" each recipient differently (Andersen, 1996). Coming to an awareness of what we do with our words and bodies to provide an intervention that fits well, can be facilitated by growing our awareness of what we actually do.

Anchoring supervisory discussions in an analysis of actual occasions of spoken and bodied interaction rather than what we "think" happens can help us notice when and how this process unfolds. This layer of examination can then be woven within broader layers construction of discourse and meaning-making. VCA enables this close analysis, moving us firmly away from a language-based, cognitive appraisal of our skills towards one which is intra-active and appraising of self in relation to the context.

The more we look in detail at our practice the more we see the minute complexity of interaction and the more we notice how tiny changes make a difference. To link with the worked example in this chapter, asking an open question to the room might be more uncomfortable to all than asking a directional question (do you know why you are here?), but it creates an early way into exploring relational patterns.

Whether a clinician is undertaking self-supervision, supervision with a peer or with a supervisor, this structured way of engaging with naturally occurring material in a supervisory context adds extra depth to reflections, and adds to the potential to develop intentional and responsive practice and to improve the communication between therapist and family. In any form of supervision, it is not necessary for the supervisor to have a training in conversation analysis, rather for them to be open to the possibility of starting with actual rather than retrospectively recalled accounts of practice.

Using VCA is not by itself a sufficient approach to supervision. The re-presentation of myself on video is a partial, situated, interpreted construction formed within the making of the material (Mondada, 2009). Words in their speaking are meaningless and need to be understood in the larger flow of living, bodily activity (Katz and Shotter, 1996). The same words uttered with the same underlying intentions can, in their speaking, call forth very different responses (Snowdon et al., 2017). As we understand how we humans intra-act with the world around us (Barad, 2007), we need to consider the holistic, global picture as well as the local-micro one. But we do have to start somewhere, to pause, punctuate, and then move the lens in and out. This contextual way of applying VCA provides a rigorous structure from which to do so.

Reflections

Since training as a clinical psychologist and then as a systemic psychotherapist, I have recorded and reviewed my work. Being able to see myself in action affords me a different perspective so as to examine and explore what I do in my moment-to-moment interactions with clients, to see how what I do affects their next move. It provides me with a window into my practice to notice what I could not when I was present within the living moment of the work. In this pandemic-influenced "new normal" of providing online therapy, I change suddenly to now regularly have an image of myself on the screen alongside the images of my clients. This new way of seeing oneself in action opens up possibilities for developing supra-vision, that VCA can explore.

I am familiar with the process of seeking consent for recording, of explaining to the family why I am recording our conversations and how it is of benefit both to me and to them. Parents and adult carers can quickly appreciate the benefit to them and to me of making and reviewing recordings. An increasingly common question from teenagers is whether their recordings will end up on social media and it is vital to explain how recordings are treated confidentially, in the same way as all medical records. Like all aspects of consent, these conversations are dynamic and need regular review. Practical, governance issues of safe storage of clinical material and the negotiation of permission to share recordings with supervisors also needs careful attention.

It has taken a long time for me to become comfortable enough with seeing myself on tape. Noticing how I fiddle with my hair, when I start and stop writing, when I sit forward or back in my seat, when I move down to sit on the floor or when I take a big breath, pause, and then shift the direction of the conversation have been painful but also useful. Noticing these things has enabled me to do more of some things and less of others.

Holding on to the memory of how anxious I felt when I first had to share recordings of my work with others (which still occasionally grips me), as a supervisor I have found that showing recordings of my own work with supervisees, modelling using the layers of context as a way of starting the discussion as shown above serves to reduce the power imbalance, to show that the anxiety of doing this is manageable and useful indeed.

A brief comment on what difference recording our work might make: while we might believe that any change to the process of doing therapy might have an impact on it (Barad, 2007; Helps, 2017), there is no solid evidence to suggest that the mere introduction of a recording device, whether audio or video, materially changes what happens in a clinical session (Speer and Hutchby, 2003; Peräkylä, 2011). However, the inherent reason for recording and reviewing work, whether as part of self-supervision or in supervision with others, is to change and improve my practice! In my own research based on video recordings of my clinical practice, I noticed that I really performed for the camera, that I tried to up my game so that what I did was the best it could be (Helps, 2019). In reflecting on what difference being a CA research made to his psychoanalytic practice, Peräkylä (2011) suggests that his many years of doing CA research did not significantly influence the way he practiced as a psychoanalyst, that is, that his extensive knowledge of CA did not sit within his reflective awareness as he chose his next move. However, he did think that his CA experience might have changed his post-hoc self-reflection and note-taking. In this vein therefore, it may be that using VCA as a supervisory tool does not change current, in the moment practice but that it enables a focussing on the small but significant ways in which interactions make a difference for the "next" session.

VCA therefore provides me with a rigorous and structured way of examining recordings of interactional practices and focusing on what I was actually doing as opposed to what I thought I was doing. Learning basic VCA transcription helped greatly with this. Although time-consuming, seeing the text and action together enabled a new perspective on the material that could then be re-connected with the video and with the broader layers of context, to make some hypotheses about the process of the clinical encounter.

I have found the use of VCA in self-supervision very useful. Within the systemic frame, not falling in love with one's hypotheses and opening space for multiple perspectives is key, so doing VCA within a peer-supervisory space, is always illuminating. It's a bit like a data analysis session that might be held between CA researchers, but where the focus is how to improve clinical practice rather than the development of CA theory.

You might think that you don't need to do painstaking and time-consuming video review and transcription to notice the subtleties of interaction that I have described in this chapter. You might think that it is really hard to justify the time that this kind of very close analysis of practice to managers, service commissioners, and others who have a call on your professional time. However, I think that the learning that comes from using this process within supervision, even once or twice a year is immense. The ripples of the learning will stay with you as you go on in your daily work, your focus can subtly change as you become more at-tuned to things that you simply didn't notice about yourself before. Human interaction is so very complicated, and we can easily fool our-selves into thinking that, in the moment, we can notice and then respond to all that is happening. You might think that you know your own practice so well that you are aware of your prejudices, assumptions, biases, habits. But I have found, from my own immersion in this work, that there is always something to learn.

Above all, using VCA reminds me of the amazing multi-layered com-plexity of social interaction. It makes me marvel at how we are ever able to put one conversational turn next to another and at the beauty of naturally occurring talk. Supra-vision, that is using video to review to explore our own clinical practice during all kinds of supervision is an accessible and mean-ingful way of engaging with this complexity.

Notes

1 This material comes from a research study (Helps 2019), in which consent was sought to use the material. Names and specific details have been changed to assure confidentiality.
2 This includes what can be seen on the tape. There are of course all sorts of other affective things happening for all the bodies in the room, but these cannot be "seen".

References

Andersen, T., 1996. Language is not innocent. In: Kaslow, F.W. (Ed.), *Handbook of Relational Diagnosis and Dysfunctional Family Patterns*. John Wiley, New York.

Anderson, T., 2013. Words – universes travelling by Tom Anderson. In: Malinen, T., Cooper, S.J., Thomas, F.N. (Eds.), *Masters of Narrative and Collaborative Therapies: The Voices of Andersen, Anderson, and White*. Routledge, New York.

Antaki, C., Wilkinson, R., 2013. Conversation analysis and the study of atypical populations. In: Sidnell, J., Stivers, T. (Eds.), *The Handbook of Conversation Analysis*. Wiley Blackwell, Chichester, UK, pp. 533–550.

Barad, K., 2007. *Meeting the Universe Halfway: Quantum Physics and the Entanglement of Matter and Meaning*. Duke University Press, Durham, N.C.

Barbetta, P., Telfener, U., 2020. The Milan Approach, History, and Evolution. Family Process. doi:10.1111/famp.12612.

Benwell, B., McCreaddie, M., 2016. Keeping "small talk" small in health-care encounters: negotiating the boundaries between on- and off-task talk. *Research on Language and Social Interaction* 49 (3), 258–271.

Bond, S., 2016. Supervision as a cluster of conversations. In: Bownas, J., Fredman, G. (Eds.), *Working with Embodiment in Supervision*. Routledge, Abingdon, pp. 49–79.

Bownas, J., Fredman, G., 2016. Introduction: Bringing our bodies to supervision. In: Bownas, J., Fredman, G. (Eds.), *Working with Embodiment in Supervision*. Routledge, Abingdon, pp. 17–32.

Burnham, J., 2012. Developments in social GRRRAAACCEEESSS: Visible–Invisible and voiced–Unvoiced. In: Krause, I.B. (Ed.), *Culture and Reflexivity in Systemic Psychotherapy*. Abingdon, Routledge, pp. 139–160.

Chodoff, P., 1972. Supervision of psychotherapy with videotape: Pros and cons. *American Journal of Psychiatry* 128 (7), 819–823.

Cronen, V.E., Chen, V., Pearce, W.B., 1988. Coordinated management of meaning: A critical theory. *Theories in Intercultural Communication* 66–98.

Doak, L., 2019. "But I'd rather have raisins!": Exploring a hybridized approach to multimodal interaction in the case of a minimally verbal child with autism. *Qualitative Research* 19 (1), 30–54.

Erickson, F., 2011. Uses of video in social research: a brief history. *International Journal of Social Research Methodology* 14 (3), 179–189.

Fruggeri, L., 2018. Different levels of analysis in the supervisory process. In: Campbell, D., Mason, B. (Eds.), *Perspectives on Supervision*. Routledge, London, pp. 3–20.

Gale, J., Newfield, N., 1992. A conversation analysis of a solution-focused marital therapy session. *Journal of Marital and Family Therapy* 18 (2), 153–165.

Goodwin, M.H., Cekaite, A., 2018. *Embodied Family Choreography: Practices of Control, Care, and Mundane Creativity*. Routledge, Abington, OX.

Helps, S., 2017. The ethics of researching one's own practice. *Journal of Family Therapy* 39 (3), 348–365.

Helps, S.L., 2019. Exploring first conversations with children and families: Responsive, pivoting improvisation within systemically-informed practice. Doctoral thesis, 2019, University of Bedfordshire. Retrieved from: https://uobrep. openrepository.com/bitstream/handle/10547/624009/Repository%20HELPS %20Sarah.pdf?sequence.

Jefferson, G., 1988. On the sequential organization of troubles-talk in ordinary conversation. *Social Problems* 35 (4), 418–441.

Katz, A.M., Shotter, J., 1996. Hearing the patient's 'voice': Toward a social poetics in diagnostic interviews. *Social Science and Medicine* 43 (6), 919–931.

Kramer, J.R., Reitz, M., 1980. Using video playback to train family therapists. *Family Process* 19 (2), 145–150.

Kykyri, V.L., Karvonen, A., Wahlström, J., Kaartinen, J., Penttonen, M., Seikkula, J., 2017. Soft Prosody and embodied attunement in therapeutic interaction: A multimethod case study of a moment of change. *Journal of Constructivist Psychology* 30 (3), 211–234.

Lee, V., 2018. The organisation of access in child mental health assessments: a conversation analysis of initial assessment appointments at a child and adolescent mental service. https://lra.le.ac.uk/handle/2381/42786 (accessed 29.11.2018).

McQuown, N.A. (Ed.), 1971 The Natural History of an Interview. Microfilm Collection of Manuscripts on Cultural Anthropology, XV (95). University of Chicago Library, Chicago. https://www.lib.uchicago.edu/mca/mca-15-098.pdf (accessed 09.11.2020).

Mehrabian, A., 1972. *Nonverbal Communication*. Routledge, New York.

Mondada, L., 2009. Video recording practices and the reflexive constitution of the interactional order: Some systematic uses of the split-screen technique. *Human Studies* 32 (1), 67–99.

Nevile, M., 2015. The embodied turn in research on language and social interaction. *Research on Language and Social Interaction* 48 (2), 121–151.

O'Reilly, M., Karim, K., Stafford, V., Hutchby, I., 2015. Identifying the interactional processes in the first assessments in child mental health. *Child and Adolescent Mental Health* 20 (4), 195–201.

O'Reilly, M., Kiyimba, N., Lester, J.N., 2018. Discursive psychology as a method of analysis for the study of couple and family therapy. *Journal of Marital and Family Therapy* 44 (3), 409–425.

O'Reilly, M., Lester, J.N., Muskett, T., 2016. Children's claims to knowledge regarding their mental health experiences and practitioners' negotiation of the problem. *Patient Education and Counseling* 99 (6), 905–910.

O'Reilly, M., Parker, N., 2013. "You can take a horse to water but you can't make it drink": exploring children's engagement and resistance in family therapy. *Contemporary Family Therapy* 35 (3), 491–507.

Pearce, W.B., 2006. Doing research from the perspective of the coordinated management of meaning (CMM). Available from https://www.taosinstitute.net/Websites/taos/files/Content/5692988/Overview_of_CMM_in_Research_version_2.0.pdf (accessed 27.12.18).

Peräkylä, A., 2011. A psychoanalyst's reflection on conversation analysis's contribution to his own therapeutic talk. In: Antaki, C. (Ed.), Applied Conversation Analysis. Palgrave MacMillan, London, pp. 222–242.

Psathas, G., 1992. The study of extended sequences: The case of the garden lesson. In: Watson, G., Seiler, R. (Eds.), *Text in Context: Contributions to Ethnomethodology*. SAGE, Newbury Park, pp. 99–122.

Ray, W.A., Saxon, W.W., 1992. Nonconfrontive use of video playback to promote change in brief family therapy. *Journal of Marital and Family Therapy* 18 (1), 63–69.

Rober, P., von Eesbeek, D., Elliot, R., 2006. Talking about violence: A microanalysis of narrative processes in a family therapy session. *Journal of Marital and Family Therapy* 32 (3), 313–328.

Scaife, J., 2009. Use of recordings and other technologies in supervision. In: Scaife, J., Scaife, J. (Eds.), *Supervision in Clinical Practice: A Practioner's Guide* (second ed.). Routledge, London, pp. 221–241.

Shotter, J., 2007. Not to forget Tom Andersen's way of being Tom Andersen: the importance of what "just happens" to us. *Human Systems: The Journal of Systemic Consultation & Management* 18, 15–28.

Snowdon, D.A., Leggat, S.G., Taylor, N.F., 2017. Does clinical supervision of healthcare professionals improve effectiveness of care and patient experience? A systematic review. *BMC Health Services Research* 17 (1), doi:10.1186/s12913-017-2739-5.

Speer, S.A., Hutchby, I., 2003. From ethics to analytics: Aspects of participants' orientations to the presence and relevance of recording devices. *Sociology* 37 (2), 315–337.

Strong, T., Busch, R., Couture, S., 2008. Conversational evidence in therapeutic dialogue. *Journal of Marital and Family Therapy* 34 (3), 388–405. doi:10.1111/j. 1752-0606.2008.00079.x.

Watson, R., 2018. Jointly created authority: A conversation analysis of how power is managed by parents and systemic psychotherapists in children's social care. *Journal of Family Therapy*. https://doi.org/10.1111/1467-6427.12244

Wilkins, D., Lynch, A., & Antonopoulou, V. (2018). A golden thread? The relationship between supervision, practice, and family engagement in child and family social work. Child & Family Social Work, 23(3), 494–503.

Wilkinson, R. , 2014. Intervening with conversation analysis in speech and language therapy: Improving aphasic conversation. *Research on Language and Social Interaction* 47 (3) , 219–238.

Chapter 14

Communication in research, evaluation, or audit

Tania Hart and Gillian Eccles

Introduction

There is a wealth of evidence highlighting the importance of research that aims to get a better understanding of children and young people's life experiences, perspectives, values, standpoints, developmental needs, and life trajectories. All of this is supported by the United Nations Convention on the Rights of the Child, 1989 (Office of the United Nations High Commissioner for Human Rights), which stipulates, children globally have the right to express their views on matters that impact their lives. Often the broader goal of conducting a child-centred research enquiry is to seek new or more accurate information about children and their experiences, as they themselves perceive them. Such knowledge has the potential to inform a wide array of child-centred local, national, and global policies and practices because it enables adults to better understand, engage, and support the needs of children.

It is fair to say that in health and social care it is now common practice to involve children and young people in research, as well as other forms of enquiry, such as service evaluations and clinical audits. This information has important value because it can potentially make a difference to children's lives by, for instance, helping to develop health related policy or cutting-edge clinical interventions and therapies as well as improving and assuring the quality of everyday intervention and practice. A classic example of an historical piece of research having great influential power on national policy, even today, is Bowlby and Robertson's (1952) child-focused investigation, whereby the findings underpin the rationale for parental open visitation rights to visit their sick child in hospital. This recommendation being derived from their films, whereby they observed the potentially detrimental effects of hospital stays on young children.

Carrying out research with children and young people does, however, have challenges; a major one being effectively engaging with the young person on an interpersonal level and getting the communication right, especially considering the imposed generation gap between child and adult. It is therefore imperative, in order to maximize the research time spent with young people, that great attention is paid to one's own interpersonal skills, how you communicate and the language you use (O'Reilly and Parker, 2014). This applies to both quantitative and qualitative researchers, auditors, and those involved in service evaluation activity. This is because communication in research is often all encompassing, involving written or verbal communication which often seeks to engage communities, as well as individuals. It is also fair to say communication is needed at every stage in the research process, whether it be in the preliminary stages of data collecting or at closing when disseminating the research findings. Furthermore, sensitive, in-depth, qualitative enquiry also requires the researcher to possess more advanced communication skills as it is crucial to engage with a vulnerable young person effectively and safely.

This chapter aims to provide those interested in child-focussed enquiry with some helpful engagement and communication tips. We first distinguish research communication from everyday professional communication. Then we introduce the reader to some commonly adopted child research communication strategies. We then highlight the benefits of improving our research communications by consulting and involving children and young people more proactively in our research projects as well as highlight the importance of using creative mediums to promote research engagement and communication. Throughout this chapter we detail and share some of our own research experiences, when carrying out different forms of child-focussed research.

How research-focussed communication differs from other forms of professional communication

Before we move onto discuss communications in research, it is useful at this point to outline the similarities as well as the major differences between other forms of professional communication, that maybe, clinical, recovery-, or formulation-focussed communication, or conversations that take place in the teaching arena, whereby they revolve around pedagogic or pastoral supports. The communication approaches used when carrying out these differing types of professional communications, to some degree, like research communication, all share a common objective, which is to sensitively enquire and evoke information, whereby the young person feels able to share their personal information. To gain an individual's trust just like all other professional communication, research communication is also underpinned by Rogerian principles of congruence (being genuine and real) and unconditional positive regard (being non-judgmental, respectful, and accepting) (McLeod, 2019).

Despite the similarities of research and other enquiring professional conversations and communications, they do however differ. Very importantly, research-based conversations aim in the main (not in all cases) to remain neutral as the goal is to gather new or more up-to-date information without making judgements or without influencing the data or outcome. Very often there is no emphasis (except for research methods like clinical trial interventions) on striving for therapeutic benefit (Targum, 2011).

Those professionals trained in differing forms of interviewing will need to separate clearly their routine professional roles from their research role. Remembering that the objective of research-focussed conversation is in the majority of cases, not to offer therapy, support, or help, but to ensure, within the parameters of the research project, the young person(s) have their say about the issues that are important to them. Upholding this neutral stance can pose the researcher, who is more accustomed to facilitating therapeutic or supportive interventions, with a challenge. As senior CAMHS professionals we have frequently found ourselves shuffling our clinical and researcher hats and so over the years have found ways of compartmentalizing our differing roles and maintaining neutrality. Below we outline some of our tips and reflect on how we partition our roles:

- Think carefully prior to conducting your research about the action process and signposting you will do if a child becomes distressed or needs further assistance during your research activity. This is also an ethical consideration and ensures you partition your roles.
- In your initial introductory conversation and participant information sheet, remember to outline briefly the parameters of what you can and cannot do in your role as a researcher.
- Refrain from advice giving during the interview so as not to be sidetracked away from your topic of enquiry, however, allow time following your research activity to give advice or therapeutic support or signpost information to alternative help if needed.

Gillians reflection below outlines *the importance of separating out clinical and researcher roles*

It is now common and statutory practice within CAMHS services and other agencies to evaluate clinical practice by gathering outcome information. Such practice is driven by the Child Outcomes Research Consortium (CORC) whose business it is to collate via specially developed, age appropriate measures, information from young people about their mental health service support. What I have found, over the years, is it is important to assertively boundary my psychotherapy role from my evaluator role. This ensures children can then be supported in their own transition from taking *part in therapy, to being in a more objective enabling frame of mind whereby they feel self-confident enough to autonomously fill out an evaluation questionnaire.*

Segregating one's clinical responsibilities, can however be a personal challenge. What I have found helps, is having a demarcation between therapy and evaluation activity. I do this by introducing the measures to the child before therapy begins and letting them know what I will be asking them to do in the end 5 minutes of our time together. I will then explain why the measures are needed and how they will be used. I always ensure I finish as promised. I then inform the child the therapy session is over and it is now their time to fill in the measure. I provide some explanation of how the measure will be used to inform service improvement and give instruction as to how it needs to be filled in, and always provide a caveat to the child emphasizing there is no right or wrong response to the questions. I give them the opportunity to ask any questions about the measure and if they reject the request to fill it in or are demonstrating signs of uncertainty, I then take time to explore with them the use of outcome measures and how this helps develop service provision. In most the cases the child responds well once they have an understanding of the purpose of the activity. If a child still refuses to take part in any clinical evaluation it is important to honour their decision, reassuring them that it is OK not to participate whilst being mindful of the child adult power imbalance.

As an Art Therapist I also encourage the children to decorate and personalize their questionnaires with drawing or stickers. This provides them with a degree of ownership promoting their autonomy and free thinking. I have found I sometimes have to guide the child when they ask, "How do I answer this?" I also prepare to explain and reframe any questions that the child may not understand. It is during this time, very importantly, I also need to remain cognizant of the importance of remaining neutral in my stance, avoiding influencing the answers the child provides. I have always found this purposeful partitioning of time, along with clear explanation encourages child autonomy helps me to remain neutral in my stance.

The attributes of good child- and young-people-focussed research communication

Very importantly a prerequisite of any successful research activity is effective interpersonal communication, whether it be engaging with an individual child or a group of children. Research is however often constrained by various variables that is, availability of time, finance, ethical, or safeguarding constraints, often making it challenging. The literature on child-centred research provides some helpful recommendations as to how to engage and communicate more successfully with children. Some of these recommendations, along with our own practice reflections, are themed below:

Promote understanding and respect from the outset

Before meeting your young participants, it is important to prepare to listen. Often children and young people have given up their time to talk to you and it is therefore very important not to fall into the trap of carrying out research *on* children and young people rather than *with* them (Balen et al., 2006). As an adult researcher, you can misinterpret or not comprehend properly what they said because your adult assumptions get in the way. It is widely recommended amongst those who carry out child-centred research methods to help safeguard against this phenomenon by carrying out some worthwhile preliminary re-flexive work. This involves you examining your own experience of childhood or getting in touch with the child inside you. Laws and Mann (2004) in their Save the Children toolbox recommend you spend time reflecting on your childhood (which is never an easy task the older you get). Ask yourself how you as a child established your trust in an adult. For instance you may ask yourself any of these questions:

- What components of this adult's persona promoted two-way adult/child conversation? Or indeed prevented adult/child conversations?
- If two-way conversations were promoted, what components of any conversation promoted it?
- Think back. What made you feel happy to share your point of view and trust this adult in these instances.
- What has made you hesitant in the past to share anything with an adult?

This type of preliminary reflective exercise aims to help you better engage with your young participants, as you are more likely to adopt some of the identified helping attributes, which promotes careful listening, enabling you to make fewer assumptions.

It is also important at the outset of the study that the adult researcher thinks very carefully about how they will equalise the power dynamic between themselves and the young person to promote better interpersonal engagement. It is therefore important you do not perceive yourself as the expert, as this is an "adultist" attitude which risks hampering engagement and may prevent you from obtaining valid and reliable data. A good tip is to ensure every young participant is made to feel like the "expert", as this in itself helps to balance the asymmetrical power dynamic. Freeman and Mathison (2009) suggests the researchers should introduce themselves to the child using their first name and reframe from the use of titles; the rationale being it goes someway to equalise the balance the power. We have always found it useful when engaging children in research, to say very clearly at the outset of the research activity "I am really interested in what you have to say and share, as it is your views that are important". We also emphasise to them at the outset, and remind them at appropriate intervals during the research, "There are no right or wrong answers or responses". This We have found goes some way to break down the power dynamic between an adult and child.

Setting the scene

All child-centred conversation should be conducted in a setting where the child or young person feels physically and emotionally comfortable and safe. A pleasant pre-booked, warm room with comfortable surroundings suggests to the young person that they are valued and important (O'Reilly and Dogra, 2016). In some instances, this may be the school, CAMHS, or Social Services office. Researchers tend to be divided when it comes to conducting interviews in the family home. Some saying it is not always an ideal venue, especially when discussing sensitive topics when there is a risk of interruption; however, the other school of thought is that it is best to engage children in the place they feel most relaxed in which is often the home. So, when carrying out research in the home it is important to establish there is no safeguarding concerns prior to conducting the interview and that the child feels free to be able to talk. If carrying out research in the home is deemed acceptable, be mindful of how the interview space is set out. Special attention needs to be placed on proxemics, explaining to the child again why you are there, how long you maybe there for, and what activity they will be asked to participate in. You may then negotiate with child where they would like you to sit before sitting down and where they wish to sit.

It is also important at the very beginning of any engagement with a child or a group of children that ground rules are established. For instance, when conducting a focus group, we might consider "ground rules" like respecting each other by listening, trying not to talk over each other, not making fun of each other, or not talking about what is shared in the group outside. When interviewing one child, you may agree as to what happens when there is an interruption, that is, stop conversation or carry on.

The role of nonverbal communication in building rapport

Freeman and Mathison (2009) states the effectiveness of child-focussed research conversations lie in the closeness of the interaction between researcher and their participants. What can promote this closeness is an aura of all-inclusiveness. To do this, adopt the principles of ensuring equal opportunity; valuing diversity and recognizing every child has their own unique individual story to tell. This is because children will quickly work out whether you have an interest in them or just want to extract information. Inclusiveness is best promoted via open body language, that is, smiles, eye contact, laughter (if appropriate), as well as adopting a welcome which is presented in the right tone and manner. So, for example a warm, engaged, interested researcher who introduces themselves on first-name terms might say with a smile and happy tone: "Hello Chloe, welcome, it is really good to meet you. My name is Jonathan, but you can call me Jon". Children need to see you care via your expressive body language which must not be over the top as this can risk being patronizing. It is also important to remember that body language can give clues as to the researcher's level of comfort and competence. Children and teenagers, like adults, tend to be very attentive to non-verbal communication and it is these non-verbal cues that can have an impact on the way they perceive their role in the researching process and the relationship they then adopt with you in that process.

Appropriate humour and laughter are also important because it can break down many barriers and promote engagement with children. It is useful to ask yourself, prior to engaging with your young participants, how you may in your professional role appropriately share a sense of fun and humour when engaging with them.

Promoting enquiry and asking the questions

Formulating the right questions, considering the child's development age and understanding, is especially important when undertaking qualitative research with children and to some degree must also be considered when developing closed- and open-ended survey questions for quantitative research with children. A rule of thumb when undertaking a child-centred enquiry is only ask young people/children questions that they can answer from their own experience. So, do not, for instance, ask them about nature walks unless they have experienced a nature walk. An important point to remember is that unlike many adults, younger children tend to live in the present and are less pre-occupied with the past or the future. Try to incorporate the flexibility into your question cue or prompt sheet that encourages them to talk about their everyday lives, allowing them (considering the parameters of your research) to have the flexibility to talk about what matters to them. So, think twice (and reflexively) about adopting a very structured question technique for interview or focus groups. Good interview cue sheets should identify broad areas for discussion with some prompt questions if needed, but it should not be a battery of questions which make the young people feel interrogated or tested because they feel the need to give the "right" answers. The aim is to encourage open discussion with both boys and girls which facilitates the process of them sharing the reality of their lives, in their way, and from their perspective.

When questions are asked it is important to be prepared to phrase your questions in lots of different ways, just in case the child does not comprehend your question or its focus. Remember also that what one child understanding won't be what another understands, so be versatile in finding ways of saying the same thing. If using questionnaires, pilot or trial them with children of the same age, prior to using them real time. This ensures the language and the way the question is structured is comprehendible to the child group you are targeting. Tania witnessed a very good example of the need to do this, when sitting in a school reception listening to two young boys around 11 years of age completing a questionnaire together. One boy read one of the questions out aloud: "What do you need to be a good listener?" They paused, then the other boy said, "I know, ears". They then moved on to the next question. She was sure that was not the information the questionnaire designer desired!

In most cases, the right open-ended questions will encourage the right feedback. My tips being move away from using "how" and "why" questions all the time, but try to use the child's words to frame your next question. For example: Raj, a young participant, says: "attending the stress management group at CAMHS really helps me to relax". The Researcher replies: "Tell me Raj how does the stress management group help you do that?". Indeed, research has shown that using the child's own words, for example with a "you said x" preface does encourage elaboration (see Karim et al., this volume; Kiyimba et al., this volume).

Also, do not be afraid to use affirming statements supporting their strengths so for instance you may ask questions like: "So that was brave, what did you do next?" "That's sounds like you did well there Tell me more". It is very important, however, not to ask leading questions as these have no place in research. For example, questions such as "What are you feeling, confusion?" run the risk of diluting your data as they may influence the child's response.

It may be more appropriate when enquiring into a sensitive topic to step carefully making sure a child feels comfortable answering your questions. In some situations, you might use third-person questions, that is, "What do you think other children would say about …", or "What do you think your best friend might say to this question …". Third-party questions often feel less intrusive than more directed personal questions and it is surprising how quickly young people move from third-party discussion to speaking about themselves.

Using reflective statements

Active listening is paramount to effectively engage. This is done by listening carefully to what the child or young person has to say as well as conveying via open body language and spoken language that you have heard and understand. Active listening can promote the child's feeling of comfort and a sense that what they are saying is valued. This then provides them with a sense of confidence enabling them to continue expressing their own opinions and perceptions. In order to ensure correct interpretation, it is always important when communicating with children to seek additional clarification whenever necessary and reflect or summarise their response to confirm accuracy. This sends a very clear message to your young participant that you have heard. The below examples are taken directly from a one to one interview with a young participant who was sharing some sensitive information related to her mental health (anxiety and obsessional compulsive behaviour disorder (OCD)). She was describing a difficult school experience associated with it. It was, therefore, important to keep the neutral researcher focus but also convey empathy. You will notice questions are not used; however, reflection is used and acts as an enquiring tool as she soon went on to elaborate on her experience:

Young Person:

"Yer. because in science classes when we have done an experiment even if it is nothing to do with chemicals I still have to wash my hands and my teacher will get cross with me and she will say oh fine you will not do another exam, another experiment next time, I am like … coz I was fussing, I was worried about getting things on my hands and I made them sore".

Researcher:

"She didn't understand about you needing to wash your hands".

This reflection, concisely summed up her feeling – note no question was asked; however, the child choose to tell me more about the difficult question.

Young Person:

"Yer I shouted at her in front of the whole class because I was so stressed and I said I have got OCD I can't help it. She was like OCD is not that much of a problem, not a problem really. Then I got moved because I was being fidgety and noisy in class and everything because I was clicking my pen because it keeps me distracted concentrating and this other girl was getting annoyed with me and she started yelling at me and then I got moved".

Researcher:

"It sounded like you were having a difficult time with your OCD and not being understood and when people do not have any understanding, it sounds like it can be very tough".

This was a more complex reflection, summarizing what she had said but conveyed empathy. Once again, no questions were asked but the child went onto tell me more.

Young Person:

"The teachers even asked my mum if she had got information about OCD, she said no she hadn't, I am not sure, it could be, quite rude to ask that because you should know about it already ... but yer ... bad".

The importance of consulting with children throughout the researching process

Plenty of evidence has emerged over the last decade that emphasizes the importance of involving children and young people more directly in the research process, whereby research philosophies that are more interactive than extractive are being more frequently promoted. This emphasis means that young participants have more of an equal role to play in making decisions about their treatment, rather than passively following the recommendations made by their mental health professional, all of which has driven improvement and innovation in children and young people's mental health provision. For instance, in the mental health field, the DOH in 2015 made history by not only listening to children and young people's experiences of their mental healthcare but also summarizing their opinions in the Future in Mind (DOH, 2015) policy document. Never before have children and young people been so centrally involved in driving forward such important strategic policy in child mental health. Another good example of this type of child involvement in the mental health arena is the "CYP-IAPT Learning Collaborative" which provides children and young people with an opportunity to be involved in participation groups that enable them to give feedback on their experience of using services via participation groups.

Considering the above, it is important when carrying out child-centred research to consider how you may involve children more proactively in your research. There is no one right way to involve them, however it is important to ensure their role is one of "active" participation. This might mean consulting and working alongside them at various points in the researching process. A seminal model proposed by Sherry Arnstein, back in 1969, "A Ladder of Citizen Participation", proposed ways of ensuring adult citizen involvement in planning processes. This seminal work has since been adapted by Hart in 1992, whereby he more directly linked it to school pupil participation in research. It is now a tool well utilized by child-focussed researchers. Based on rungs of a ladder, it outlines the various levels at which young people can actively participate in research.

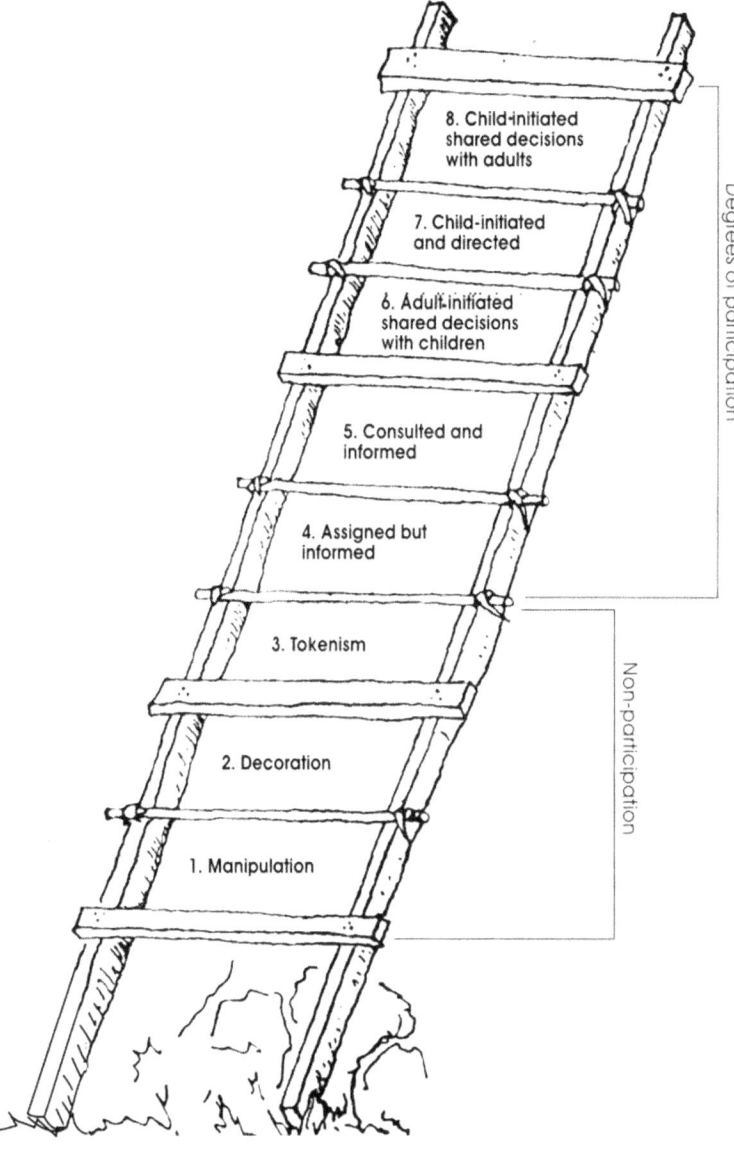

Figure 14.1 Adaption of Hart's ladder (1992, p. 8).

It may not be feasible for researchers to be able to get to rung 7 or 8 because of research methodology or ethical implications; however, whatever your form of enquiry you can try to ensure you have listened and involved young people in the planning or reviewing of your research (rungs 5 and 6). This is because the more discretion young people can exercise over the content and direction of the project, the more likely the research conducted will reflect their true views; for instance, consulting with children about interview research questions will ensure the questions that are asked matter to children and children see the point in answering them. Tania's reflection below demonstrates this:

Reflection: The power of participation I was project leading an evaluation of a city whole-school resiliency promotion programme, whereby various new strategies had been introduced into schools to promote pupil well-being and resiliency from classroom activity looking to promote emotional and digital literacy to parenting support groups. Our task as evaluators was to evaluate impact.

As often is the case, we were financially restrained and working to meet a dictated deadline. Our project would not allow us to reach 7 or 8 of the participation ladder, however to ensure the right data was captured, we undertook some important preparatory discussions. Whereby we consulted and listened to young people from similar age groups and backgrounds as the children who were to participate in our research (ladder rung 5). This phase of consultation enabled us to better develop and adapt our questionnaires and interview guides, thus ensuring our survey tool would be fit for purpose suiting the various populations of school children from those in key stages 1 and 2 and the needs of children who did not speak English.

It was surprising how much useful information the children gave us. For example we learnt that some of the pictures or stories we wanted to include in our questionnaire, that made sense to us, made no sense to them. They also provided us with better ways to engage their peers with the questionnaire exercise, by suggesting teachers should not just give pupils the questionnaire because they felt their peers would not see why it should be completed. They suggested the questionnaire filling should follow a fun class activity around emotions. So, we developed short lesson activities considering their recommendations; for key stage 2 we developed a word search activity linked to an emoji PowerPoints game. It was interesting to find that the schools that incorporated the additional activity had fewer defaced or blank questionnaires. So, the children were correct!

The consultation group also advised us to change some of the words on our questionnaire and include short vignettes to promote comprehension (see fig 14.2 below that illustrates how one question was framed using a vignette (other questions followed on from this one).

One of the children in your class is brand new to the school. You notice they are finding it difficult to make friends. Think about your feeling and behaviour in this situation, would you:			
	No	Sometimes	Yes
25. Try to be nice to others because you **care about** their **feelings**.			

Figure 14.2 Children's feelings question from the STRENGTHS AND DIFFICULTIES QUESTIONNAIRE (SDQ) S11-17 adapted by T Hart to include a vingette to promote understanding.

Using creative mediums in research to promote engagement and communication

Many qualitative researchers carrying out child focussed enquiry such as, focus groups, interviews, or a range of other participatory methods, often incorporate creative methods like drawing, playdough, puppets, Lego, music, etc., or possibly technological media's like photography and video. This is because research communication can be enhanced with children when structured around several activities (Castro, Swauger, and Harger, 2017), the benefit being it helps young participants remain engaged and on task with the enquiry in hand. A variety of techniques can prevent boredom and sustains interest. Having something specific to respond to also helps the young person who struggles with concentration (i.e., those with attention or concentration difficulties), enabling them to make connections with the topic of enquiry.

Playful and creative approaches can be especially useful when carrying out a sensitive line of enquiry whereby difficult feelings are likely to be expressed. Creative activity in these cases can be helpful because the child can talk about something else rather than themselves enabling them to more safely externalise their difficulties. Therefore helping to keep the conversation light and playful as this reduces stress and provides children with an opportunity to bring their own distinctive contribution.

A word of caution however when embracing the concept of using creative activity you must firstly ask yourself, do the creative methods truly have a place in supporting your line of enquiry, and are you sure you are not hiding any adult insecurities behind such structured activities?

When creative mediums are felt to be appropriate to promote communication and engagement with children researchers must consider the development and holistic needs of the child. A piece of seminal work carried out by Rhoda Kellogg between 1948 through 1966 tells us that researchers need to also consider the child's artistic development. Rhoda, a psychologist and a director of a nursery school in San Francisco, examined the development of artistry by collecting over one million drawings from children of different ages. She then categorized these into developmental stages, as outlined below:

- **The Scribbling Stage** ages 2–4 – This is random mark making.
- **The Pre-schematic Stage** ages 4–7 – This is where the child begins to name their scribbles.
- **The Schematic Stage** ages 7–9 – The child represents a real object, creating symbols that can be simple or really intricate. The child is representing their own artistic vision.
- **The Dawning Realism Stage** ages 9–11 – The child becomes aware of their art making and begins to judge it. They will be interested in others and are aware of their peers and society.
- **The Pseudo-Naturalistic Stage** ages 11–13 – There is more of an emphasis on the end product, being aware of their own artistic talent and having phases of creativity.

It is helpful to remember that once a child has reached school age, they will more frequently question their wider world and their place in it and might look to you for more guidance and ideas. Therefore, it is important to have this in mind that is, if a child asks a question like: "What do you think about heaven"? The appropriate response would be to encourage the child's wondering. So, for example, you respond with "I am not a heaven expert, but what do you know and think about this and what are your thoughts and feelings?"

Once a child moves into the teenage years, self-criticism and the idea of artistic talent being something they do or don't possess will be in-built. Hence, using creative mediums is different to engaging younger participants. It is necessary therefore to think carefully about the methods you will use. Ask yourself, does the activity have potential to patronise? Crayons and paints may make some teenagers feel like children if the activity is not age appropriate. Drawing is, however, appropriate when the activity is age appropriate for example. Gauntlett (2007) asked teenagers to draw pictures of celebrities to understand their aspirations and their identifications with media figures. Varied and imaginative research methods such as vignettes (short stories), YouTube clips, or photos work well with older children, as does incorporating internet, mobile phone, or webcam activities. This is because many young people are very used to being bombarded with vibrant, fast-moving visual pictures and the downloading of photos and videos onto social media via Apps such as WhatsApp and TikTok. Researchers have found these mediums to be less intimidating than asking teenage participates to wholly participate in a one-to-one interview. Media such as film clips and photos have been seen to promote a relaxed atmosphere, appearing to increase the young people's confidence whilst being interviewed (Punch, 2006).

A useful reflexive exercise to do when looking to use or develop creative activities to promote your research communication is to take the time to watch children or young people in your targeted age play or engage in leisure activity. Ask yourself the following questions: What are they doing or playing with? Who are they playing with? What makes the activity fun?

Gillians reflection below outlines the power of creative medium, not only enabling successfully engagement with a vulnerable young person, who spoke little English, in therapy but also how evaluation of this intervention could be carried out neutrally and sensitively via pictures and scales.

Reflection: The power of art as a medium to cross language barriers and when carrying out sensitive enquiry

I was working with an unaccompanied asylum seeker, also known as a separated child (as this term places the child first), who had faced many traumas in his war-torn country. His mother had paid traffickers to get him safety to this country but when making this journey he had experienced more trauma. He presented with post-traumatic stress disorder and he was having flashbacks to the traumatic incident.

I often used art to engage and communicate with him, as his interpreter was not always available. He would use the art materials to draw images of his village, family, and friends. He drew a picture of a boat which depicted how the boat had been attacked and had sank. This drawing invited me into his experience. Although we could not communicate, he knew certain words and I could empathise through facial expressions and making my own artwork in response to his painful traumatic experience. This reciprocal art making became the conversation. I also used emojis that depicted differing facial expressions for him to rate how he was feeling during the session which helped me gauge his emotions when I was uncertain.

To gain feedback from the session. I used a session-by-session rating scale with a line divided into green amber and red that ran from the thumb's up to the thumb's down. This method helped to evaluate our trauma work.

Reflective practice piece

Our top tip is to prepare well before engaging directly with any young person in your research and think carefully about how you are going to engage and interact with them. The reason being, when carrying out your actual research it can often be too late to make corrections or adjustments and research time with children is often precious. Therefore, time spent consulting with children prior to commencement of your research is time well spent, as is time piloting or testing your interview questions or tools.

Tania's reflective piece below intends to combine many of the points discussed in this chapter. It describes a study whereby teenagers with diagnosed emotional problems were interviewed, the aim being to explore how they perceived they could be better supported at school. The reflection outlines Tania's experiences of carrying out this preliminary work with children from consultation, tool development, and piloting.

Reflection: The importance of prior preparation

I only had forty-five minutes with each of my participants. I had to maximise my time with them, ensuring my semi-structured interview were planned down to the tee. My problem was I did not have the privilege to have met the young people before they were interviewed, therefore faced the challenge of having to build a relationship with them quite quickly in order that they felt at ease talking about the sensitive topic of mental health.

Preparation was key. Due to the sensitive nature of my enquiry, I decided not to rely solely on direct questions. Subsequently I developed some film clip vignettes which could be drawn upon as needed to engage and promote conversation. These clips depicted various school scenarios and were written and coproduced by children from a local drama group. They were short 2-minute clips depicting different named characters experiencing mental health difficulties at school and who were dealing with common school scenarios i.e., classroom learning activity, common peer and teacher interactions, etc.

Once these films were developed, I took the time to consult with another group of teenage children and asked them what they thought of our film clips and interview questions. They advised me to show the film clip vignettes on an iPad only when needed and to keep to broad questions as they felt many children their age would happily talk about their school experiences because it was a matter that concerned them.

Following on from this consultation, I undertook some pilot interviews with teenage children who did not have a mental health problem. These pilots enabled me to refine my interview skills yet further in that they highlighted some of my bad communication habits like falling into the trap of asking leading questions, therefore allowing me to rectify this. When I did eventually interview my young research participants, I found they had no problem talking to me. I felt confident and came away with some rich data. However, the prior preparation I am sure helped.

Conclusion

Carrying out child-centred research enquiry in its many forms, from surveys too interviews, can be challenging because ultimately it is about ensuring children feel confident enough to want to tell you about their experiences and perceptions. Think carefully about how you may engage and communicate with your young participants, considering their unique situations as well as their developmental age. This will ensure you can adapt and strengthen your communication style accordingly. To summarise, then, we offer some practical tips in Box 14.1.

Box 14.1 Practical tips

Practical tips for improving communication

- When asking questions, refrain from making it like an interrogation, weave your young participant's words into your next question.
- Be mindful of the power imbalance between child and adult researcher and ensure every stage of the research process is collaborative and transparent.
- Pay particular attention to preparing the scene; the environment, organising resources, setting the rules and the boundaries.
- Ensure, within the scope of your research, that the children have the flexibility to talk about what matters to them, ensuring they do the majority of the talking.
- Refrain from asking leading questions; they have no role in the research process.
- Reflecting back what the child has said has its place in research interviewing. It can be helpful because it demonstrates active listening and can build empathy and trust.
- Develop appropriate creative mediums, considering the child's age, to promote engagement and communication.

References

Arnstein, S.R., 1969. A ladder of citizen participation. *Journal of the American Planning Association* 35 (4), 216–224.

Balen, R., Blyth, E., Clabretto, H., Fraser, C., Horrocks, C., Manby, M., 2006. Involving children in health and social research "human becomings" or "active beings?" *Childhood* 13 (1), 29–48.

Bowlby, J., Robertson, J., 1952. A 2-year-old goes to hospital. *Proceedings of the Royal Society of Medicine* 46, 425–427.

Castro, I.E., Swauger, M., Harger, B., 2017. *Researching Children and Youth: Methodological Issues, Strategies, and Innovations* (first ed.). Emerald Publishing Limited, Bingley, UK.

Department of Health, 2015. Future in Mind: Promoting, Protecting and Improving Our Children And Young People's Mental Health And Well-Being. NHS England Publication Gateway Ref. No 02939. linkhttps://assets.publishing.service.gov.uk/government/uploads/system/uploads/attachment_data/file/414024/Childrens_Mental_Health.pdf (accessed 21.11.2020).

Freeman, M., Mathison, S., 2009. *Researching Children's Experiences.* Guildford Press, The USA.

Goodman, R., 2001. Psychometric properties of the strengths and difficulties questionnaire. *Journal of the American Academy of Child and Adolescent Psychiatry* 40 (40), 1337–1345.

Gauntlett, D., 2007. *Creative Explorations: New Approaches to Identities and Audiences.* Routledge, London, United Kingdom.

Hart, R.A., 1992. Children's Participation: From Tokenism to Citizenship. In: Innocenti Essay, vol. 4. International Child Development Centre, Florence.

Laws, S. Mann, G., 2004 So you want to involve children in research? A toolkit supporting children's meaningful and ethical participation in research relating to violence against children. https://www.savethechildren.org.uk/content/dam/global/reports/education-and-child-protection/so-you-want-to-involve-children-in-research.pdf (accessed 29.1.2020).

McLeod, S., 2019. Person centered therapy. https://www.simplypsychology.org/client-centred-therapy.html (accessed 09.11.2020).

O'Reilly, M., Dogra, N., 2016. *Interviewing Children and Young People for Research.* SAGE, London.

O'Reilly, M., Parker, N., 2014. *Doing Mental Health Research with Children and Adolescents: A Guide to Qualitative Methods.* SAGE, London.

O'Reilly, M., Ronzoni, P., Dogra, N., 2013. *Research with Children: Theory and Practice.* SAGE, London.

Punch, S., 2006. Interviewing strategies with young people: The "secret box", stimulus material and task-based activities. *Children & Society* 16 (1), 45–56.

Targum, S.D., 2011. The distinction between clinical and research interviews in psychiatry. *Innovations in Clinical Neuroscience* 8 (3), 40–44.

Index

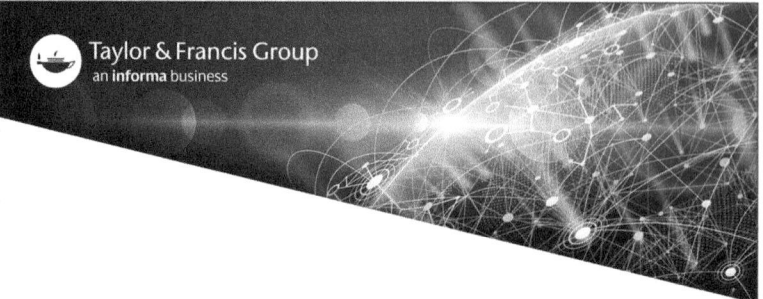
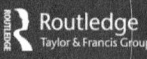
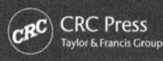